RUNNING WITH NATURE

Stepping Into the Life
You Were Meant to Live

MARIEL HEMINGWAY
and BOBBY WILLIAMS

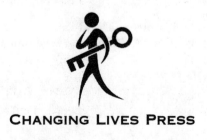

CHANGING LIVES PRESS

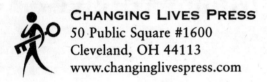

CHANGING LIVES PRESS
50 Public Square #1600
Cleveland, OH 44113
www.changinglivespress.com

Library of Congress Cataloging-in-Publication Data is available through the Library of Congress.

ISBN-13: 978-0-9882476-1-1

Editor: Lisa Espinoza
Cover photo of Mariel and Bobby by David Paul
Cover and Interior design: Gary A. Rosenberg • www.thebookcouple.com

Printed in the United States of America

10 9 8 7 6 5 4 3 2 1

CONTENTS

*We dedicate this book to NATURE
and all the beauty, knowledge and
simplicity it offers all of us daily.*

ACKNOWLEDGMENTS

May the sun always shine on all our amazing friends and, of course, our family Paul, Joan, Janice Williams and John Boddy, and Dree and Langley Hemingway for their radiant support of this passion project.

Cheers to Heather Reinhardt for her patience and sweet attitude toward our process; Karyn Dilworth for keeping the faith; Dan Horton, Lisa Erspamer, Tara Sheahan, and David Paul who are extended family; Joe Kolkowitz (without whom Bobby would not have written this book), all of whom inspired us to keep going; and Barbara Kopple for introducing us to our wonderful publishers Ellen Ratner and Francesca Minerva.

Thank you to those who always saw and continue to see the vision: Mike Call, Boone Speed, Nancy Lee, the Hubtuit team, Chris Montgomery, Brian Mezner, Melissa Beaver, Karen Baxter, Tracy Columbus, Kevin Desoto, Jen Ward, Ian Clark, Ryan Culver, Jim Crabbe, Brett Fairall, Jon and Andrea Benson, Victoria Diiorio, Stefanie Hartman, Tania Hartman, Scott Paton, Alix Thelemaque, Josh and Selene Carmichael, Cathy and Dayne Seiling, Jim and Alexis Kwik, Marty Davis and Cambria, Asher and Alice Milgrom, Steve Oates, Andy Langberg, Kevin Fortun and Robert Heggie at Mariel's Kitchen group, Mike and Joy Van Noy, Craig Kessler, Rachel Goldstein, Lori Hart, Dr. Thai, David Thorson and Fairway.

Thank you Alan Hopkins and Paul Sears for keeping the Running With Nature Ranch alive. Thank you Margot Dougherty for organizing our initial thoughts, and finally Lisa Espinoza, our editor, who saw this project through to the end. We are profoundly grateful to all of you!

Bindu, Lucy, Tree, Mow and the ladies (hens)—Thank you for your fur, your feathers, your eggs and wags. . . . WE LOVE YOU.

INTRODUCTION

WELCOME to *Running with Nature!* Life on your own terms.

As we both thrive at 50, we are finding that the impossible is becoming possible. It really is possible to be younger, happier and healthier than ever before. Our motto is live your life and forget your age. We believe that age is more about habits, choices and lifestyle than about the number of years gone by. We have only been on this earth about 18,250 days (50 years) so far. A short time in the giant scheme of things, don't you think? Every day is a new beginning. And remember, the sun shines for us all with each new day. We are alive and vital and as young as we feel—and we feel incredible, ebullient, vibrant and free. How about you?

The common belief is that we're all supposed to retire at 65. Our life expectancy is 75, and disease and overall degeneration will do us in. Really? There's no way we're buying into that. We are here to let you know that we will all break these rules together. We plan on living many more adventurous days on this planet. How about 73,000 of them? Or more? Is it possible? Why not?!

Each day we are given 24 hours. That's 86,400 moments to change our lives for the better. We are here to inspire you to use the gift of each moment to become the best teacher, healer, nutritionist, trainer and guide *to yourself* that you can be. How can you do this? By becoming an expert in being YOU! Now, in this moment. And the next, and the next, and the next. Learn to be your authentic Self by taking actions that are natural, doable and accessible—watch a sunrise or sunset, drink pure water out of a glass, take time to be silent, eat clean food, and take a step back from technology. As you will find, the single action that reenergizes us the most is getting outside and connecting with Nature by doing something physically and mentally challenging.

Running with Nature is more than a book—it is a lifestyle. Each of the ten chapters that follow focuses on an aspect of living that is vital to our well-being. As you read, you'll notice that we're continuously exploring the male/female dynamic, the yin/yang, or the balance of relationship if you will. So together and individually we talk about how to get the best sleep, eat the best foods, drink the best water, and finally how to breathe (as simple as it sounds, how we breathe is a powerful and complex tool). And let's not forget the importance of being playful and having fun.

Point-Earning Activities Checklists

Our goal is to inspire and motivate you to make the Running with Nature lifestyle changes that will result in a healthier, more vital You. We also give you the tools to make this happen. At the end of each chapter, we provide you with a list of Point-Earning Activities that will help you put into practice the ideas you're learning about. Choose *at least one* activity per chapter every day to enhance and expand your life and help you grow into the Running with Nature lifestyle.

This is not a strict point system but rather a practical guideline for incorporating healthy new choices into your everyday life. Think of your points earned or lost as energy. Assuming you've given yourself a good night's sleep, you will wake up with 100 points. Earn 100 more points in a day and you've gained a day's worth of vital life energy! You can gain points based on the simple choices you make throughout the day. Awareness is the key. Make it your intention to do those things that are going to add to, not subtract from, your health and well-being. Your goal is to earn as many points as you can—Running with Nature points are life-giving points! There are limitless possibilities for Point-Earning (i.e., life-giving!) Activities that are playful and feel like things you *get* to do rather than *have* to do.

Point-Earning Activities, those we've listed or the ones you come up with yourself, will increase your positive energy and result in greater health than ever before. Of course, we can't promise you extra days, but we can promise you this—all you need is the will, and you will find your way to your greatest life.

Invite Others to Join the Journey

Once you begin practicing the Running with Nature lifestyle and experiencing the benefits firsthand, we are sure that you will want to share it with friends, family and others. You may consider starting a Running with Nature group that gets together to talk about how you are incorporating the Running with Nature ideas for living your best life and to share ideas for more innovative Point-Earning Activities.

If you like competition, challenge one another to earn the most bonus points by engaging in additional healthy activities above and beyond the ones suggested in each chapter. The winner gets a prize in keeping with the Running with Nature lifestyle—no, not a case of Budweiser, but maybe a week's worth of green juice from the local health store, a massage, a new bike, or a new kettlebell! You could also meet at the local farmers market or get together for a long hike, a picnic or a neighborhood block party. Imagine a Running with Nature community that inspires and supports one another on the journey toward greater health and vitality!

Whether you embark on this adventure alone, as a couple or with a group of friends, the key is to make this shift in lifestyle fun and positive. Believe us when we say that Running with Nature is about living your life and having fun doing it.

Tune In to YOU!

In this book, our goal is to help you tune in to yourself. This will not only shift your own state of mind, it will also benefit your relationships with your partner, your family, your kids, your colleagues and, by extension, the world. Becoming conscious of the simple things you do in life will help you to become more present and will connect you to a greater self-awareness. The human trinity of body-mind-spirit has the ability to accomplish greatness, to be extraordinary.

Many of us have allowed ourselves to become disconnected from the simple things that keep us grounded and healthy. Do you race through your life missing the moments that count? Do you feel you're just too busy to slow down, to take a deep breath and connect with your own inner place of peace and calm? We call this connection being centered. We'll show you how to stay centered even in the midst of this crazy world we all live in. Take a journey of discovery and learn the tools to be the greatest *You* that you can be by making simple yet powerful daily choices. It really is within you to take charge of your life by consciously choosing each day how to live it.

People often say we live an "alternative" lifestyle. This simply isn't true. The real "alternative" lifestyle consists of eating processed, pasteurized, synthetic, radiated and genetically modified foods, drinking alcohol, caffeine, and sugar water, watching hours and hours of television, and never turning off the computer or other electronics. That is an alternative lifestyle. The very *real* and very *conscious* lifestyle that Nature intended all along is what *Running with Nature* is all about . . . a simple lifestyle in tune with Nature's rhythm.

Not so long ago, people lived off the land. They performed physical labor and connected to their families and friends, building a strong sense of community. Most of today's society is living disconnected from Nature. We know how easy it is to buy into the convenience of microwave ovens, fast food, technology and too little sleep. We've lived that life, and we won't go back. For us, turning away from constant convenience and tuning in to the simplicity of Nature became the key to joy, health and vitality. It can be the same for you.

In the following ten chapters, we'll show you how to be a part of this modern world without allowing it to compromise your immune system and rule your life. You will learn how to become a teacher and a guide of your own existence by slowing down enough to create time and listen to your inner Self. We will help you to reconnect to your authentic Self and absorb its vibrant energy. In the process, you will feel younger and regain a childlike curiosity that fills every day with wonder.

Each of us possesses our own unique way of connecting with our Self. Ours may not look like yours. We cleanse by fasting. We plunge into icy mountain streams and dive into the ocean in mid-winter. We ride motorcycles through the desert and climb 1,000-foot rock faces. Our adventures make us present and mindful. They create balance in our body, mind and spirit. They give us joy and make our lives rich. Now as we share our experience, we hope that you will be inspired to find your own unique ways of living an amazing life.

All of us face the big questions of life at some point: *Who am I? Why am I here? What moves me? What are my dreams? Who do I want to become in this moment? How can I leave this place better than I found it?* They can be answered by the everyday choices you make in food, thought, breath, exercise, stillness, Nature and adventure. Although we are extreme in some of our choices, we encourage you to find your own pace for change. If you want to improve your diet, start with eating a healthier breakfast, or try one new healthy food each week. If you prefer to dive in headfirst, go for it. You can overhaul the way you eat right now—this minute!

If you want to meet your Self through adventure, step further into the unknown and try something that stretches you more and may even fulfill a secret desire: kayaking, dancing, singing, mountain biking or surfing—anything outside your comfort zone. The most challenging experiences in life are the ones that let us know we are alive. They awaken us to our greatest potential.

Your journey is your own. We're here to encourage you to break free from the one-size-fits-all mentality in your approach to life. We want to give you the information to explore and find your own path with confidence. We are here to help you find who You are now, in this moment, by connecting you to your true nature through the purest of teachers: your TRUE Self. Everything you ever need to know is within you.

For us, Nature is everything. It is true simplicity. It is truth, without ego or agenda. The power of Nature connects us all. Nature was, is, and always will be here now. It surrounds us and is within us. The simplicity of being outside and feeling the earth beneath our feet makes us more us. The wind itself carries messages. Stop, listen, and feel the energy run through your body and know that it runs through all of us.

We enjoy living a life of curiosity. We continually ask the question, "Who am I being right now?" That always brings us back to the beginning, the present moment. A person who thrives in life is healthy, connected, mindful and present. You can become aware of how best to heal your body simply by knowing that *you can* in any given moment. You are much more powerful than you realize.

Join us on our journey from morning to night. We'll share our day's first thoughts with you, our first words, our first movements and our pilgrimages into the wild. We'll help you understand how a decision you make in one area of your life will affect another—what you eat for breakfast affects what you eat for lunch and how you will feel throughout your day. You may find that making a ritual of your morning tea or juice is a simple but transformative action. As you begin to experience the Running with Nature lifestyle through the daily Point-Earning Activities, you will discover your path to a younger, healthier, happier You.

The road less traveled isn't a road at all. It is a path that you create for your own personal journey as you find a lifestyle that works for you. The world is without boundaries—be the orchestrator of your own life simply because you can. All it takes is willingness. Use this book with the realization that you are bringing to light your innate ability to be extraordinary.

> *"Nothing is original. Steal from anywhere that resonates with inspiration or fuels your imagination. Devour old films, new films, music, books, paintings, photographs, poems, dreams, random conversations, architecture, bridges, street signs, trees, clouds, bodies of water, light and shadows. Select only things to steal from that speak directly to your soul. If you do this, your work (and theft) will be authentic. Authenticity is invaluable; originality is nonexistent. And don't bother concealing your thievery—celebrate it if you feel like it. In any case, always remember what Jean-Luc Goddard said: 'It's not where you take things from, it's where you take them to.'"*
>
> —JIM JARMUSCH

Running with Nature is simple and accessible—real food, clean living, a clean environment, knowing where your food and water come from, connection to the planet and the world of Nature, conscious physical movement, silence and listening within. All of these things will help you to know yourself. Where there is a will, there is a way. This is the Running with Nature philosophy. Let's get started!

CHAPTER 1

GET OUTSIDE

"It is very simple to be happy, but it is very difficult to be simple."

—RABINDRANATH TAGORE

Our connection to Nature is innately our connection with ourselves because we are inherently Nature. Whether it's your backyard, Yosemite, a local park or the Amazon rainforest, we believe it is about breaking free from "the matrix." In the iconic movie, characters had to choose between the blue pill (representing the blissful ignorance of illusion) and the red pill (representing the sometimes painful truth of reality). We all wake up each day faced with the same choice. We strive to choose the red pill often in our everyday lives by connecting to those things that are real and inspiring. We're talking about mountains, rivers, oceans, forests, dirt—the ground from which everything else rises. Nature predates us and, unless we are so negligent as to destroy it, will endure long after we are gone. Nature is life's constant, connecting us with our ancestral roots and with all the generations to come. Nature is never-ending and always beginning.

Spending time in Nature helps us unplug from the urgency of technology and to-do lists and plug into our true Selves. It gives us the space to remember who we are without all the socially defining and confining stuff like cars, schedules and professions defining us by what we have rather than who we are. When we put ourselves in settings dominated by natural forces and primordial order rather than by man's interpretation of time, we have a chance to feel a universal connection. We can remember the simplicity involved in leading lives of freedom, happiness and compassion.

Mariel: I have always believed that God and Nature are somehow intertwined. I believe that Nature gives us instructions for how to be happy and well—how to be the best that we can be. Since I was a child, I have always been happiest outside—breathing clean air, challenging my body to go beyond what it feels it can, climbing to a mountaintop and looking out over the vista. Whether it is in Sun Valley atop the ski slope, beneath a waterfall in Big Sur, or next to the cliffs that jut out of the ocean at Big Rock, to me, God lives in Nature. Bobby feels the same. Nature connects us to who we are.

Bobby: Words pale in comparison to the reality of the rugged mountains, endless oceans and vast deserts of the great outdoors. Living the experience is the understanding—discovering otherworldly cloud formations folding on summits and crevasses so deep they seem to go on forever; drinking ice cold glacial water; watching lightning rip through the sky; observing satellites as they creep across the moon; feeling the power of the ocean as you ride the waves and paddle with the dolphins. I once had the tail of a whale slap down ten feet from me. I stared in awe and remembered how small I actually was.

I love this place! There aren't enough hours in the day to see all there is to see. The great news is I get to do it again tomorrow. Nature is a great metaphor for life because Nature is never ending and always beginning.

Aside from being wondrous, Nature is infinitely practical. Trees and forests are our planet's lungs, absorbing the carbon dioxide we produce. The Indians say that the trees are our closest relatives. There is no more intimate relationship than this—what we breathe out, they breathe in, and vice versa. Everything we need for survival—food, water, air, sunlight, shade, medicinal remedies—comes from Mother Earth.

The numbers and statistics from the Amazon rainforest alone are staggering and impressive. Also known as the lungs of the planet, more than 25 percent of the world's oxygen and 80+ percent of the world's diet is derived from the rainforest. Countless holistic and traditional medicines have been used to heal people for thousands of years. Three thousand fruits are found in the rainforest. While only 200 of these are now used in the Western world, the Indians of the rainforest use 2,000. Over 28 billion gallons of water flow from the Amazon River into the Atlantic every minute. And yet, well-known environmentalist Al Gore has verified that we are eradicating rainforests at the rate of a football field per second. While you are reading this sentence, a few more football fields worth of rainforest are disappearing.

> *"When the last tree is cut, the last river is poisoned,*
> *and the last fish dead, we will discover that we cannot eat money."*
> —NATIVE AMERICAN SAYING

Nature is the muse of scientists as they seek ways to imitate its genius. The Biomimicry Institute in Montana is devoted to adapting Nature's designs to human endeavors. By studying an African beetle, the institute developed a mechanism for pulling moisture from the air and used it to create a water system for humans. Canadian-based Nexia Biotechnologies looked to the process of spiders spinning their webs as a basis for the manufacture of BioSteel, a substance that, pound for pound, is five times stronger than steel. The company hopes to use the material to produce bulletproof vests and medical equipment. Ford's Volvo Division has developed an anticollision system based on the way locusts swarm without crashing into one another. IBM studied the formation of abalone shells as a template for making computer processors. As we said, Nature is brilliant. When we work with Nature instead of against it, we can be brilliant too.

The following is based on a letter sent by the Pennsylvania Department of Environmental Quality to a man regarding a pond on his property. The man's response is hilarious, but read the State's letter before you get to the response. This is an example of how far we have drifted from working with Nature and appreciating its innate genius.

SUBJECT: DEQ File No.97-59-0023; T11N; R10W, Sec. 20; Lycoming County

Dear Mr. Smith:

It has come to the attention of the Department of Environmental Quality that there has been recent unauthorized activity on the above referenced parcel of property. You have been certified as the legal landowner and/or contractor who did the following unauthorized activity: Construction and maintenance of two wood debris dams across the outlet stream of Spring Pond.

A permit must be issued prior to the start of this type of activity. A review of the department's files shows that no permits have been issued. Therefore, the Department has determined that this activity is in violation of Part 301, Inland Lakes and Streams, of the Natural Resource and Environmental Protection Act, Act 451 of the Public Acts of 1994, being sections 324.30101 to 324.30113 of the Compiled Laws, annotated.

Sincerely,

David Jones, District Representative

Land and Water Management Division

Mr. Jones' response:

Dear Mr. Jones,

Your certified letter dated 12/17/02 has been handed to me to respond to. I am the legal landowner but not the Contractor of the dams. A couple of beavers are in the process of constructing and maintaining two wood "debris" dams across the outlet stream of my Spring Pond.

While I did not pay for, authorize, nor supervise their dam project, I think they would be highly offended that you call their skillful use of nature's building materials "debris." I would like to see your department attempt to emulate their dam project any time and/or any place.

My first question to you is: (1) Are you trying to discriminate against my Spring Pond Beavers, or (2) Do you require all beavers throughout this state to conform to said dam request? If you are not discriminating against these particular beavers, through the Freedom of Information Act, I request completed copies of all those other applicable beaver dam permits that have been issued.

I have several concerns. My first concern is—aren't the beavers entitled to legal representation? The Spring Pond Beavers are financially destitute and are unable to pay for said representation—so the State will have to provide them with a dam lawyer.

Being unable to comply with your request, and being unable to contact you on your dam answering machine, I am sending this response to your dam office.

Thank You.
Mr. Smith and the Dam Beavers

Escape the Craziness

Did you know that according to Nielsen Company researchers, the average American watches more than 4 hours of television a day? They say by the age of 65, we've spent 9 years parked in front of the TV. Herbalist Dr. Richard Schulze estimates the number as high as 15 years! We figure that if you add an extra 3 hours on Saturday and another 3 hours on Sunday for sporting events (such as football games —both college and NFL, the NBA, college basketball and March Madness, baseball, golf, tennis, NASCAR), that totals over 20 years! Imagine staring at a box for 20 years. When you're 65 years old, will you be satisfied knowing you've spent 20 years of your life watching other people live their lives on TV instead of really living your own? Wouldn't you rather spend that 20 years doing all the things you love, learning and discovering the wonderful experiences real life has to offer? Sure makes you think, doesn't it? So what's it going to be— 20 years of sitting or 20 years of living?

We live in a rustic getaway in Southern California, surrounded by mountains and just a short drive to the beach. When day-to-day stresses of life start mounting, Nature is our means of escaping the craziness and stepping off the treadmill for a while. We often disappear into the mountains behind our house, surrounding ourselves with negative ions—molecular particles of energy that are believed to produce biochemical reactions that increase serotonin levels, which can help to alleviate depression, relieve stress and boost our daytime energy. These negative ions are present in abundance in natural settings such as mountains, waterfalls and beaches.

One of our favorite pastimes is road-tripping into the outdoors. We've found unbelievable hot springs, 14,000-foot peaks, waterfalls 8,000 feet up, and cold plunges. The greatest thing for us is always the silence, which is extremely difficult to find in a world that moves so quickly.

Sometimes we'll be in a place so quiet, the only sound we'll hear is the sound of our own breath. We love being completely off the grid in places where no one has stepped before, so far from civilization that not even a plane interrupts the tranquility—like parts of the Sierra National Park that are no-fly zones. In this silence, we gain perspective on life. We get up when the sun rises and go to bed when the sun sets. We eat when we're hungry. We don't have a care in the world, and time doesn't exist. There is only the present moment.

In this quiet place, the noise of our minds is cleared away, and the stillness creates space for us to just be. This is exactly why Nature is such a powerful tool in helping us remember who we truly are. Nature just is. The sun just is. It cannot be made less real. The more experiences we have with things that are real, the less false we become. So it's all about stripping away those things that are not really us—the chemicals, the toxins, the negative thoughts, the busyness, the mind chatter, the distractions, the stimulants . . . the noise in all its various forms.

> *If you listen:*
> *Nothing in nature lives for itself*
> *The rivers do not drink their own water*
> *The trees do not eat their own fruit*
> *The sun does not give heat for itself*
> *The flowers do not spread fragrance for themselves. . . .*
> *The connection is one living organism . . . Nature*

When we experience this reality—this authenticity of who we are—we are more accepting of ourselves. We stop looking outside of ourselves for approval, and we start to focus on the meaning of our lives. Why are we here? Where are we going? What can we contribute to ourselves and to others? It's a connection that starts with us and overflows into the community and the world around us. The result is that we stop habitually following others and start leading ourselves.

Who Are You?

Wouldn't it be amazing to live up to *your own* unique potential? Too often people put themselves in a box dictated by their family, education, religion or society at large. But what's the purpose of being like somebody else? How about finding out who *you* are? Step outside the box. Connect with what is real and you will experience tremendous personal growth. You will discover your own individuality and perhaps your life's purpose.

> *Bobby: When I take people climbing, they usually have a lot of fears in the beginning. I'll tell them to put their right hand at "2 o'clock" and they immediately look to do something with their left hand. I say, "No, your other right hand," sometimes two or three times. It stops them from moving forward. It stops them from listening. The mental adrenaline compromises their ability to think clearly. Working through this fear brings change and a deeper understanding of themselves. This same fear shows up in their everyday walking around life too. When we have this fear, we stop listening. We stop being ourselves.*
>
> *Failures can be glorious achievements when we get up again and again knowing that we gave it everything we had—win, lose or draw. These are the defining moments of our lives and when we are at our best!*

Nature presents us with endless opportunities to learn who we really are and to overcome our fears. Ask yourself, "What can I do to step outside of myself to create change and growth?" When we allow Nature to teach us, we move through fear and grow in the knowledge of ourselves, and this newfound confidence is carried over into every area of our lives.

Walk Barefoot

"The best runner leaves no tracks."

—TAO TE CHING

Walking barefoot is natural. It is something that has been done for thousands of years. We believe it's become a lost art and is something we should all do more of—allowing the soles of our bare feet to connect to the earth and in turn to connect back with ourselves.

In *Born to Run*, Christopher McDougall talks about the lost art of running. He tells the story of the Tarahumara tribe of Indians in the Copper Canyons of northwestern Mexico, a group of people known for their amazing ability to run hundreds of miles without rest or injury, usually barefoot or wearing the thinnest of homemade sandals. From the Tarahumara tribe, McDougall learned that we were all born to run—because we run.

> *Bobby: Running is one of our greatest gifts. Learning how to run is a metaphor for life. I love to run! In the book* Born to Run, *Christopher McDougall speaks of flipping an internal switch that changes us all back to the natural born runners we once were— not just in history but in our own lifetimes. Remember? Back when we were all kids, we were always yelled at to slow down! Every game and sport was at top speed. Half the fun of doing anything was doing it at record pace—taking the chance that this might be the last time in your life you would ever be hassled for going too fast.*
>
> *Running was mankind's first fine art, an original act of inspiration. Distance running was revered because it was indispensible. It was the way we survived and thrived to cross the planet. You ran to eat and to avoid being eaten. You ran to find a mate and to impress her, then you ran off with her to start a new life together. You had to love running or you wouldn't live to love anything else.* Born to Run *reminds us that we were born to run simply because we run.*

Some friends from CrossFit asked us if we had noticed that running shoes were on a diet, slimming down thanks to the popularity of *Born to Run*. It's interesting that we're going back to our roots. Walking or running barefoot on the beach, on a hiking trail, or even in your backyard or a local park can be invigorating. You may think, "My feet will get dirty!" Exactly. When we walk barefoot, we allow ourselves to connect with the energy of the earth's electromagnetic field—we become grounded. According to many Eastern traditions, the earth's energy pushes through the feet and into the body's 12 main energy pathways, called meridians, helping to rebalance the body. This is why the ancient practice of yoga, indoors or out, is done barefoot.

When your bare soles connect with the pure earth or sand, you receive the free gift of energy right beneath them. How simple and transformative is that? Remember to start slowly and choose wisely when finding places to walk or run barefoot, and be aware of any potential dangers. We highly recommend you choose your own backyard, a pristine park, a wildlife area or hiking trails in your neighborhood that you are familiar with. Territory with which you are unfamiliar may pose dangers due to topography, insects or other wildlife, or even the soil itself, which may contain harmful bacteria. Also, be sure that you start slowly to acclimate yourself to this new way of connecting with Nature. Be particularly careful if you are overweight—you may want to limit your barefoot walking to flat ground or the harder beach to minimize the possibility of taking a fall.

Mariel: Nature is powerful. Whenever I'm in the ocean, I feel the excitement of knowing it has the power to crush me. But there is also a paradoxical feeling of ease in knowing that my ego has been put squarely in its place. Nature is BIG. Its grandeur is spectacular. Humanity seems miniscule in comparison. Nature brings me back to center. When the stresses of life start mounting, Bobby and I go outside. He goes climbing, or if he feels really out of balance, he goes off into the Sierras for a few days to reconnect himself to himself by himself. I stay home and go out for hours into the local mountains. I stay away from technology. When I get really quiet, I am able to reconnect with me.

Bobby: When you find yourself in challenging situations out in Nature, it's either thrive or simply survive. In these situations, awareness is heightened as we find ourselves present in the moment. A sense of well-being awakens, and we remember who we are and who we can be. There is a powerful feeling that anything is possible. For me, this is what it means to be "in the zone." I get to this quiet place in my mind and my body, and instead of giving in to panic, everything slows down and all that I do becomes effortless, almost surreal. Whether I'm surfing or climbing, running or walking, or quietly sitting in these wild places, there's a strong sense of knowing, seeing and being. I know who I am and I am home.

When you place yourself in challenging situations and emerge safely, your confidence and awareness increases. You come away with a sense of well-being and of being able to take care of yourself. The same inner strength that moved you to explore the crags and crevices of the mountain will follow you into your classroom, your corporate job, your relationships—into every part of your everyday life.

Here Comes the Sun

"Here comes the sun . . ."

—GEORGE HARRISON, 9-26-69 • THE BEATLES, ABBEY ROAD

The sun is our source of boundless energy all day. It brings us warmth, light and life. There are so many reasons to embrace the sun. It demands our attention, for it is the largest star in our solar system. It feeds plants that absorb light energy to make food. A plant is always reaching up toward the sun, never sideways, always up. It is quite a powerful principle if you think about it. Like the plants that derive life from the sun, we too yearn for the sun and yet have forgotten how much we need it. We would do well to mimic the plants and reach for the sun to absorb its energy and vitality.

We absorb the sun's energy by sungazing, sunbathing (natural sunscreen in place during the midday) and simply being outside.

In a sense, we are all children of the light, and hiding from it or being without enough sunlight brings both physical and emotional imbalance.

Without the sun, there would be no life on the planet.

The sun elevates our mood. Its rays enhance the effects of serotonin, a neurotransmitter that makes us feel happy. You have probably heard of seasonal affective disorder (SAD)—episodes of depression that occur certain times of the year, particularly during the winter months. The cause of SAD is thought to be overproduction of melatonin, a hormone that our brains produce during times of darkness. When the hours of darkness lengthen, some of us produce an excess of melatonin, which can lead to depression and irritability. When springtime arrives, those with SAD find themselves back on track in terms of their mood. For those sensitive to the lack of light, making a point of getting outside during sunlight hours is especially important.

Although viewing the sun during an eclipse can be harmful, moderate sungazing as the sun rises and sets is generally considered safe. We've been bombarded with warnings about how damaging unprotected sun exposure can be, but our bodies need those solar rays to produce vitamin D. This vitamin is essential for maintaining proper levels of calcium and phosphorus, which are critical for bone health. Vitamin D also helps to keep our immune system functioning properly. According to the Mayo Clinic, vitamin D may help protect against osteoporosis, high blood pressure, cancer and some autoimmune diseases. Dr. Andrew Weil recommends moderate sun exposure, about 15 to 30 minutes without sunscreen at least twice weekly, to help our bodies produce vitamin D in sufficient quantities to do their job.

The safest exposure time is in the morning and late afternoon when the sun is less intense. The two of us get our sun from between 7 a.m. and about 10 a.m. and then from 5 p.m. to the sunset hour. When we are outside during midday, we use natural skincare products like the zinc-based sunscreen from ANU Wisdom and John Masters Organics. Of course, hats and rash guards (typically worn by surfers and volleyball players) are the best protection, providing solid coverage.

We love to get up at sunrise. We go outside in our bare feet and ground ourselves through the touch of the earth as the sun makes its way over the horizon. Seeing the break of dawn, watching the world go from dark to light, and catching those first rays has such a powerful effect on us. We can feel the energy being infused into our body, mind and spirit.

The last light—sunset—is transformational too. If you get quiet and still, you feel like you're absorbing the energy as the sun fades from view. If you're lucky, you may see a green flash just before the sun disappears, an optical illusion resulting from the sun's rays refracting through the thicker atmosphere near the horizon. For a fascinating look at the ancient practice of sungazing, check out the documentary *Eat the Sun,* directed by Peter Sorcher.

We all know that the sun is the engine of photosynthesis, the process by which plants survive. Hiran Ratan Manek, better known as HRM, is testament to the empowering potential of the sun for humans. Born in India in 1937, HRM claims to have been living on little more than the sun and water since 1995, with occasional sustenance from tea, milk and buttermilk. On three occasions, he has conducted long-term fasts, abetted by solar gazing, under the auspices of medical staffs in India and the United States. According to subsequent reports, HRM is able to get all his vital nutrients through the sun. You can read more about HRM on nutritionist Dr. Joseph Mercola's website (www.mercola.com). While we certainly admire HRM, we simply love food way too much to survive on sunlight anytime soon!

The simplest path to finding and reconnecting with You is to get outside—soak in the sun, breathe in the fresh air, feel the earth beneath your feet. We'll talk about exercising in Chapter 9, but for now just get outside and enjoy everything Nature has to offer. Connect to the powerful energy of the earth, and remember that you are part of it.

POINT-EARNING ACTIVITIES CHECKLIST

GET OUTSIDE

- In the morning, before work, go to a place where there is dirt, plants, and/or trees and a sense of Nature. Leave your technology at home and take a walk (barefoot if you can), find a seat or just stand and observe your surroundings. For at least 15 minutes, forget about your agenda and appreciate the quiet miracles around you. Listen, smell, breathe.   **10 POINTS**

- Catch a sunrise or sunset.   **10 POINTS**

- In the early morning or an hour or two before sunset, spend 10 to 15 minutes in the sunlight without sunscreen. Be grateful for the easy access to vitamin D.   **10 POINTS**

- Take a conscious walk on the beach, a rural trail, or anywhere that you can enjoy the serenity and solitude of Nature. Try to keep your mind empty of day-to-day concerns and use the experience to refresh your senses and renew your awareness.   **10 POINTS**

- Climb a tree.   **10 POINTS**

- Take a leisurely swim in a lake or spring. An outdoor pool will work if you don't live near a natural body of water.   **10 POINTS**

- Geography and weather permitting, plunge into the ocean and ride a few waves.   **10 POINTS**

- Find an easy bike route that runs through a natural setting. The point here isn't the exercise (although that's a bonus); it's to find quiet and peace.   **10 POINTS**

- If you have access to a row boat, canoe or kayak, slipping through placid waters is another beautiful way to get in touch with Nature and yourself.   **10 POINTS**

- Tend your yard or garden. Deadheading roses (removing their spent blossoms), raising vegetables, and planting or tending to anything in the earth brings us directly into contact with Nature's transformative power. Live in the city? Try a potted garden on your patio or an herb garden in your kitchen.   **10 POINTS**

                              TOTAL POINTS _____

CHAPTER 2

SLEEP WELL

How much do you sleep every night? When was the last time you had a good night's sleep? Do you think you don't need much sleep? We live in a 24/7 society (cable TV, Internet, cell phones, constant communication), so indeed how we live is affecting how we sleep. According to a United States Centers for Disease Control (CDC) report, 40.6 million American adults are sleeping six or less hours a night. Too much caffeine, nicotine and alcohol compound the problem. We'd like you to consider your sleep habits in a different way than you may have up until now.

Our sleep needs change throughout the various stages of life. Infants need at least 16 hours a day, toddlers 12 to 14 hours, and teenagers 10 hours (the National Sleep Foundation reports that 50% of American teenagers are not getting enough sleep during the school year). Adults need 8 hours of sleep, but we like to get 9 depending on our activity level. We'd like to think we are successfully multiplying our productivity by having more waking hours, but when we pare down the amount of time we give our bodies to rest, we suffer significant consequences.

Sleep is a necessary time of rejuvenation. On a cellular level, our bodies are repairing and regenerating during sleep. Because children are constantly growing, developing and playing, getting enough sleep is essential to replenish their energy for all they do. We feel younger because we sleep like kids, getting sufficient sleep to keep our energy levels equal to the demands of our busy lifestyle. Honoring our body's need for sleep is an important step toward greater health, vitality and longevity.

Consequences of Lack of Sleep

Did you know that lack of sleep can tip the scale in the wrong direction? A recent study found that those who sleep 4 hours a night or less are 73 percent more likely to be obese. This makes sense—people working on too little sleep are likely to eat more snacks, most of them high in carbs and sugar. Insufficient sleep also slows the metabolism. Getting more sleep is a good way to tip the scales in your favor—literally.

Mental focus is also impacted by too-little sleep. We become ineffective in our thinking, emotionally unstable and reactive. Lack of sleep can harm our work performance, our communications and our relationships. We are likely to make poor decisions because we just don't have the clarity of mind to think things through reasonably. The irony, of course, is that oftentimes we think we're sharp—especially if we've tried to make up for sleep loss with caffeine. This overconfidence in our ability to function on sleep deprivation can lead to serious consequences. The National Highway Traffic Safety Administration conservatively estimates that 100,000 police-reported crashes are the direct result of driver fatigue each year. This results in an estimated 1,550 deaths, 71,000 injuries, and $12.5 billion in monetary losses.

Bobby: I did some extreme things in my career as a stuntman and athlete. Sometimes I'd get up at 3 a.m. and work until the last light. On one commercial, I remember a helicopter dropping me off on a 6,000-foot mesa. Between climbing, pendulum swings, high falls, and a 400-foot Tyrolean traverse, by the third 16-hour day, mistakes began to happen. The entire crew was exhausted. A producer fell on black ice and broke a leg. I sprained an ankle. To finish the job, I had to be taped up every day and could barely walk. We all learned that it makes no sense to push yourself to go without sleep to the point that you start mentally or physically breaking down. It's just not worth the risk.

Honoring Your Circadian Rhythm

The body's natural time clock is pretty ingenious. It's called the circadian rhythm. Taking its cue from light, our circadian rhythm helps regulate virtually all the body's functions. When darkness comes, the brain's pineal gland begins its secretion of melatonin—"the hormone of darkness." This melatonin calms us and helps us sleep. Melatonin production spikes in the middle of the night and then lowers, letting us know when it's time to wake up. When we tinker too much with this natural rhythm by turning on lights and staying up late, we throw all sorts of cellular maintenance off schedule. Taken to an extreme, this can lead to lack of energy and depression.

While humans like to make claims that we can stay up all night, this isn't really something to brag about. Unlike nearly 70 percent of our fellow mammals, we are not nocturnal. We are meant to sleep in the dark and be up with the light. We are tricked into believing it is still daylight by lights, televisions and computers. If you make the effort to sleep and wake with the natural cycle of dark and light (we're not expecting you to go to bed at 5 p.m. come winter, but you may want to hit the hay earlier than you do in summer), you will see positive results in your health, energy and vitality.

Your Sleep Schedule

About two hours after sunset, following the rise of melatonin, the body enters a phase of increased internal activity during which the repair and restoration of your body takes place. We both notice a difference when we go to bed earlier versus later. We find that when we go to bed at 9:00 p.m., for example, and get up the next morning at 6:00 a.m., we feel energized and refreshed. But if we go to bed at midnight and get up at 9:00 a.m., even though we've experienced the same number of hours of sleep, we wake up tired. Don't just take our word for it, try it for yourself. Try the two sleep patterns we just mentioned for a couple of nights each. You will notice a difference, and hopefully you will be motivated to make it early to bed every night. There's something to be learned from the Benjamin Franklin quote, "Early to bed and early to rise makes a man healthy, wealthy and wise."

Bobby: In our society, there are lights everywhere. We are constantly exposed to light pollution. We drive around at night with headlights glaring in our eyes. The lights in our homes are on long after the sun sets. Like the glaring lights of Broadway that keep folks wide awake all night (you've heard of the "city that never sleeps"), we surround ourselves with artificial light that tricks our brains into thinking it's daylight so that we can stay up. When I guide people in the mountains, they all talk about how they stay up late and are most creative at night. They tell me that they'll never go to bed at 8 p.m. But within two to three days, they all end up wanting to go to sleep before me, every single one of them. They start to connect with the biorhythms of the earth.

Mariel: When it comes to how many hours we need to sleep at night, everybody is different. Some people are extreme, on either end of the spectrum. Bobby needs nine to ten hours, and I need about eight and feel best at nine. For me, length of sleep used to be related to my spirituality . . . I had been practicing meditation for years and thought that I needed less sleep because my meditation would make up for my lack of it. I always thought that the less I slept, the more spiritually advanced I was. I thought I was the champion on only five or six hours of sleep. I ignored the fact that I was tired a lot of the time. When Bobby and I got together, he challenged my beliefs and encouraged me to stay asleep longer. I secretly LOVED it. The difference in the way I felt and feel is huge. I also noticed that my sleep was more peaceful, and my body began to function better. I was more calm and grounded. Even the look on my face became softer.

Taking Naps

Sometimes life throws us a curve, such as a looming work deadline or a family illness, and we just cannot avoid staying up late and getting up early. During these times, the body becomes deprived of sleep. A sleep debt is created, and the body will do its best to get us to pay up. Naps are one way to balance the sleep account. An hour's nap can supplement hours of lost sleep. But be careful not to sleep too long—

lengthy naps where you enter a deep sleep can tend to leave you feeling a bit fuzzy for up to half an hour after waking. The optimum time for a nap is about 20–30 minutes. Our power nap is this—we allow 5 minutes to slip away, 20 minutes to sleep, and 5 minutes to find our way back into the day. According to the Division of Sleep Medicine at Harvard Medical School, laboratory sleep studies show that naps of 20 minutes or so can improve attention, decision-making, reaction time and manual dexterity. A short nap can give the body a reenergizing break, leaving you fully refreshed without the sleep hangover.

> *Bobby: I am always taking naps during the day. People will tease me, "What, are you getting old?" But the truth is, I've been doing this since I was a kid, and it's just what I do. The funniest part is that it doesn't matter where I am because it's such a pattern in my life. I can just stop what I'm doing and take a 20-minute nap. Whether it's a production meeting, an audition, running around town and taking care of business, I will pull into a parking lot or pull the car over, put on some music, close my eyes, and sleep for 20 minutes exactly. Everything completely shuts down.*
>
> *Some people think this is strange, but instead of reaching for a cup of coffee, I energize with a nap. Anyone can. If you have an hour for lunch, you can eat and talk for 30 minutes and then take a power nap in your car—5 to go in, 20 to sleep, 5 to come out.*
>
> *Napping isn't a new idea; it is a tradition in other parts of the world. Most European countries close down for several hours after lunch and come back rested and ready to work. While our blood sugar is crashing, taking a little nap is a healthy, natural choice and a much better idea than turning to caffeine, sugar or energy drinks. If you close your eyes even for a few minutes, take some deep breaths and relax, you'll notice a difference.*

Your Sleep Surroundings

It's essential to reach your REM sleep, the deepest dreaming stage, during the night. This is best done by sleeping in a dark, quiet place. Ideally, you want to hear nothing more than your breathing and your heartbeat. If you go to sleep with the television on, your body isn't given the opportunity to fully unwind. It's taking in that electronic energy, physically and mentally, even while you're asleep. The same is true if there is a bright light on in your room or outside your window.

We encourage you to make your sleeping space as dark as possible. Light interferes with sleep at least partly because it inhibits melatonin secretion and thus resets the biological clock. Professor of natural sciences J. Woodland Hastings has shown that even a split-second of light exposure can shift the circadian cycle of a single-celled organism by a full hour. By creating a space that is free of light and noise pollution, you are cooperating with your natural circadian rhythms to ensure restful, rejuvenating sleep.

Rarely do we experience the kind of darkness that is only possible apart from our usual power-generated environment. Once we visited a dolomite cave in the Sierras where it was so dark you couldn't see your hand in front of your face. No matter how much we looked and looked, we couldn't see anything. Nothing. And that was in the middle of the day. Never before had either of us experienced that kind of darkness or quiet. We felt a sense of calm and peace as we allowed the darkness to surround us—no distractions at all. This is the kind of environment we were meant to sleep in.

Prepare for Sleep—"The Review"

Before we go to sleep, we like to think about how we intend to wake up and what thoughts will be guiding our new day. This interlude is a powerful time for us to express our gratitude. We tell ourselves how grateful we are for the day that just occurred—certainly for all the good things that happened, but also for the lessons we learned that may have presented a challenge for us. We review all the choices we made and experiences we had in the day. This is a spiritual practice known as reflection or recapitulation, but we simply call it "the review." It is considered a form of meditation and basically entails a mental playback of the day. We recommend doing this sitting up because—that's right—if you do it lying in bed, you'll likely fall asleep!

There is no "correct" way to do the review. You can get as specific as you like in recalling the day—what you did, whom you met, what you said, how you felt, the sensations you experienced in your body, and so on. Start with your earliest memory of the day and do your best to follow each moment after that right up to the moment you're in now. Of particular value in this exercise is to assess the day's lessons, to consider things that didn't work so well and learn from them, and then to set the conscious intention to choose a better course next time. Also, think about when you felt energized and when you felt drained. These can be clues as to how you might want to invest your time tomorrow.

The review is an extremely powerful practice for furthering growth and change. It is also a crucial time for self-forgiveness. Done regularly, it will help you release old, ineffective emotional patterns. By bringing your thoughts and choices into your awareness at this special time, when your mind is sleepy and malleable, you can program yourself to change. Just imagine: if you reflect on one thing that you would like to change each day, you can address 365 issues in a year.

Remember our challenge in the beginning of *Running with Nature* —each 24-hour day presents us with the gift of 86,400 moments, each an opportunity to change our lives for the better. By investing some of your nighttime seconds in thoughtful reflection on how you would like to effect change, you're subliminally programming your psyche to act on it the next day.

Another way to look at this is that by fixing those 365 things, you prevent them from continuing to accumulate. You will stop repeating the same patterns, the same behaviors, the same thoughts, the same emotions, and the same mistakes over and over again. Too many people never grow into their potential because they rarely stop to reflect on their behavior and make the choice to behave differently. It takes consciousness, willingness and a sincere intention to change. With this kind of mindful activity, the stage is set for a fresh start in the morning, with new choices and new possibilities abounding!

As you begin to practice your nightly review, you will develop the questions that work best for you. To get you started, here are suggestions of things to think about during your review:

- What were the most fulfilling moments in your day?

- What didn't you do today that you wish you had?

- Where were you silent or critical when you could have given an encouraging word?

- Did you miss an opportunity to create good feelings in yourself or another?

- Were there instances when you were unkind to yourself in your head?

- Were there times when you insisted on being right?

- Where did you fall hook, line and sinker into old patterns that no longer serve you well?

- Which behaviors and thoughts worked best for you today?

Your review will help you become your own best therapist. You will become an expert in You. It takes discipline, but the rewards are huge. Instead of constantly distracting your mind away from yourself—by having the TV on until you fall asleep, for example—create space for yourself. Listen. Get to know You. You are worth getting to know. This is the first act in self-love—knowing that you are worth taking the time to discover. Such a simple shift in awareness will have a dramatic effect in every area of your life.

> *Bobby: My parents used to sleep with the TV on. I convinced them to make their bedroom dark and quiet, and it changed their sleep time entirely. The dark environment gave them more space to have their own thoughts, to really consider what it is they want to do, and subsequently they started doing new things. My dad's 74, and now he surfs every day, and my mom goes in the ocean. They are thrilled with the way they've been changing and are so much happier overall. It's wonderful to see.*

> *Mariel: When I started traveling with Bobby, I was in awe at the amount of time he put into making hotel rooms, tents, the back of his truck, or a guest room in someone's home into a dark sleep cave.*

Bobby: I believe the turtles have the sleep thing figured out. These fellows carry their homes on their backs. Instant darkness and silence available 24/7. It's said that Aldabra Tortoises can live over 200 years.

Mariel: But they're turtles . . .

Bobby: Exactly right—they know something. Nature's philosophy is taking the impossible and making it possible. If the turtles can go 200 years, we can go 200 years.

Mariel: I'd like to check in at 100 and see how everything looks before I move forward. Meanwhile . . . you spend almost an hour putting bedspreads, blankets, pillows, luggage, towels, socks, and hats to cover everything from TV lights and digital clocks to smoke alarms and peep holes—making the room so dark that when you wake up you walk into walls you cannot see and have forgotten they are there. All of this seemed crazy until I realized I slept so deeply and have never been more well rested in my life. Maybe you and the turtles are on to something. . . .

Wake Up Slowly With Gratitude

We recommend that you start your day slowly whenever possible. A gentle process of waking and getting up can set the tone for your entire day. And if you move too quickly—jump out of bed—you may feel dizzy or lightheaded. We recommend focusing your very first attention on connecting to and observing your body. Crinkle your toes, stretch your legs a bit, tighten your quads, stretch your arms over your head, yawn, and check in with your breathing. Massage your face, calves and feet. Do this slowly and with great awareness. Feel the sensations in each area as you gently move from sleep to wakefulness.

When you wake up this way each morning, you become better attuned to your body—from your toes up through your fingers to the top of your head. And you become more conscious of what's going on physically, emotionally and mentally. This waking awareness is the first step to entering your day fully present. If you can start with that intention right off the bat, you have a much better chance of maintaining it throughout the day.

Once your body has gently awakened, it's time to turn your attention to your first thoughts. We like to start the day in silence as much as possible. Like the night before, the most important first thoughts will be gratitude, followed by intentions for the day. Take the first five minutes of your morning to express how grateful you are to be alive, to have this new day. Next, think about what step(s) you would like to take today to validate and create a more joyful and fulfilling life. What would you like to accomplish? What would you like to do that's just for yourself today? What enriching experience would you like to have? How can you make that happen? How would you like to be today, both within yourself and with others? Do you want to feel more joy? Communicate more consciously? Laugh more? Explore Nature? Decide what attitudes and actions you'd like to take, and become the conscious creator of your life.

Starting the day grateful—for yourself, for being in your body, for having food, for your family, for your spouse and kids, for whatever you can observe as good in your life—will help you take the rest of your day in stride. Even if problems arise, you will be able to remember that they really are manageable. Difficulties won't have the same power to dominate your mental landscape. You'll be able to relegate them more accurately to the role of single notes in the symphony that is your life.

Try to find gratitude even for the things that may not be going well. This means truthfully finding the larger good in life's more distasteful or uncomfortable moments and challenges. Our greatest lessons are often learned through the situations we find most difficult. It's a wonderful achievement to be grateful for everything that comes our way. This is the ultimate in self-responsibility—knowing that whatever is happening, we have the ability to choose how we will respond to it. The choice to be grateful will directly affect the quality of your life and your level of happiness.

The truth is, we have much more power to direct our lives than we give ourselves credit for. Many people shy away from this level of responsibility, but embracing it gives us much more freedom, and with that freedom comes happiness. Instead of all the defenses and excuses you can come up with to prove that you are not to blame, imagine what you can change about a situation when you accept that you had something to do with creating it. This is empowerment! And when you start living this way, you start truly living *your* life.

> *Mariel: Just as the night before sets the stage for your first thoughts, the early morning hours create the environment in which the rest of your day unfolds. It's so important that this time be slow, quiet, peaceful. Wake up your mind and body gradually, gently. This was a new approach for me. When I first met Bobby, I used to wake up so severely. The minute my eyes would open, I would jet out of bed. Bobby taught me to wake up more methodically. It was an adjustment, but I have found that it makes me feel much more connected and brings a greater sense of calm to the start of my day.*

Planning your day has less to do with mapping out a schedule of activities than it does with having conscious intentions about the day you want to create. When you give your life this kind of thought, which we recommend at the beginning as well as at the end of the day, you program yourself to remain present and aware. This positive mindset will prevail as you take the reins of your life. You will rewrite the script and put yourself in conscious control.

Follow a Morning Ritual

Ritual is an act of self-acceptance and love; it's a practice that you give yourself each morning that validates your worth. It's a simple, clear message that says, "I like myself." Making a mindful cup of tea and honoring yourself is a very different internal experience than having that same cup of tea while rushing out the door or grabbing it on the way to work from your local Starbucks.

> *Mariel: I love ritual. For me, any act of ritual is sacred and calming. It is a way of honoring myself and becoming more aware. For*

*my morning tea, I choose leaves that have a wonderful aroma. I
use a beautiful pot and a pretty cup. I like to include elements that
engage my senses . . . smell, taste, touch, sight and sound. The
smell of the tea leaves in the canister and when the water is
poured over them as they release their fragrance is something I
look forward to because I enjoy it on so many levels. The most
important thing for me is that I do each action mindfully, from
boiling the water, to filling the pot with leaves, to slicing a lemon,
and finally sitting down on the porch with the warm cup in my
hands and taking my first sip. There is gentleness to my morning
tea ritual that adds reverence to the beginning of my day.*

Daily ritual can be a powerful way to become more conscious and
further instill that present-moment awareness as a habit. Take an
extra 10 minutes to prepare a cup of organic loose-leaf tea, or an
organic fair-trade coffee, or light a scented candle. Go outside and
inhale the fresh air into your whole body. Close your eyes and listen
to the birds and sounds of early morning while the sun warms your
face. You can turn just about any simple act into a practice of mindfulness, and it will nurture and nourish you; it will start your day off
in a positive way.

POINT-EARNING ACTIVITIES CHECKLIST

SLEEP WELL

- Eat before 7 p.m. so your body can *rest*, not spend
  time *digesting food*. You'll be fast asleep if you do.   **10 POINTS**

- Read something inspirational before you turn out
  the light.   **5 POINTS**

- Keep your bedroom dark—invest in blackout curtains
  and hide the glowing alarm clock where it can be
  heard but not seen.   **10 POINTS**

- If you live in a noisy area, use earplugs for sleep.   **5 POINTS**

- Meditate before sleep and consider your intentions
  for the next day.   **10 POINTS**

- Go through a nightly review or recapitulation of
  your day.   **10 POINTS**

- If you have trouble falling asleep, try a cup of chamomile
  or valerian root tea an hour or so before getting into
  bed. Another alternative is to take a warm bath.   **5 POINTS**

- Wake slowly and consciously, moving, stretching,
  breathing. Give yourself five minutes to get out of bed.   **10 POINTS**

- Change your sleep routine. Try going to bed 30 minutes
  earlier if you are a "night owl" and getting up earlier.
  See if this shifts your energy, your focus, your clarity. **10 POINTS**

TOTAL POINTS _____

CHAPTER 3

BREATHE CONSCIOUSLY

nhale. Exhale. Inhale. Exhale. We all do it ceaselessly, about 20,000 times a day, an average of 12–18 breaths per minute. With every deep breath we take, we charge our bodies with an electric current, our life-force energy. Breath connects us to our bodies and is one of its most powerful cleansing mechanisms, performing about 70 percent of our detoxification process. Each day our lungs breathe in between 2,100 and 2,400 gallons of air—the amount needed to oxygenate the 2,400 gallons or so of blood that is pumped through the heart daily. By taking full advantage of breathing and its many applications, we can change our mood and our energy levels and facilitate enormous changes in the way we think about everything, including ourselves.

Breath is life, and yet so many take it for granted. Most of us breathe from the chest, sucking in our abdomen on the inhale and releasing it on the exhale. Watch how a baby breathes. Their bellies expand as they take a breath in and deflate as they let the breath go. They are totally relaxed with no tension or stress. Perhaps they're onto something. While shallow breathing or "chest breathing" can lead to tension, anxiety and chronic pain, full breathing can help get rid of all those things. It's amazing how powerful something so simple can be.

Breathing exercises are also a great way to improve the symptoms of asthma, insomnia, anxiety and other stress factors. It also helps alleviate the stresses that trigger or exacerbate obsessive-compulsive disorders. How many times have you been advised to "take a deep breath" during anxiety or irritation? There's good research behind the cliché. Oxygenating our cells helps release tension and anger. It helps us think more clearly.

An Australian study showed that mild asthmatics cut down their need for fast-acting inhalers by 86 percent after just seven months of breathing exercises. In India, researchers found that people who practiced slow-breathing exercises for three months lowered their systolic and diastolic blood pressure by 11 and 7 points respectively. Ancient yogis wouldn't be surprised. They developed pranayama, the scientific study and practice of breathing, thousands of years ago. In fact, yoga postures (called asanas) were created as movements to help the breath reach different parts of the body. Many other eastern philosophies—tai chi, qigong, shaolin, even karate—use breath as a key to attaining balance of body and mind.

The power of breath is everything. It's essential for life, health and well-being. Breath is also widely considered essential for spiritual awareness. By concentrating on the breath, we can begin to sense and to eventually gain control over our nervous system. We can ultimately learn to have voluntary control over our lungs and heart, which can lead us to discover greater power over our thoughts. By controlling our thoughts, we are empowered to control the perception of our own environment.

"Life is not measured by the breaths we take,
but rather by the moments that take our breath away."

—AUTHOR UNKNOWN

Breath, Scent and Memory

It's been said that just one deep inhalation through the nose will cause 10,000 memories to arise. We've all experienced how a particular scent brings up vivid memories. Some of those will be pleasant memories and some not so pleasant. You can use your breath to reinforce happy recollections and also to dispel negative ones. When negative memories, trauma or impacts are left unattended, they can be stored in our bodies and show up as illness or pain. Breathing and smell are deeply related and connected to our emotions. A conscious and directed deep breath can give you the space to release stored memories that no longer serve you. When you inhale, imagine your breath traveling to that unpleasant memory and flooding it—see the breath as light or color, whatever you imagine that will enable you to connect your breath to the memory. Consider the memory as you inhale, and release it as you exhale. There is no correct length of time to engage in your breathing exercise. You may need to repeat several sessions before you find that you have completely released the negative energy connected to a particular memory.

> *Mariel: Smelling the sweetness of night-blooming jasmine reminds me of a time when I was a child. I was making a movie called* Lipstick in California, *and my mother was with me. We were staying at a friend's ranch, and in the evenings the jasmine floated in the air so strongly it filled me with a peace and happiness—something I was not accustomed to because at that time my mother was terminally sick with cancer, and I had always felt responsible for her. For years afterward, I associated the smell of jasmine with my mother's illness as well as that special time. Whenever this bittersweet scent was around, it put me into a place where I felt guilty over being happy, healthy and alive. Over time, I came to recognize this pattern and released it. Now I can smell night-blooming jasmine, and it reminds me of how much I loved my mom.*

Breath and Healing

Conscious inhalation, breathing deeply into the lungs, can bring healing energy into the body and its organs. Long, deliberate exhales expel toxins and help your body get rid of things you don't need. On a spiritual level, this type of intentional breathing helps connect you to yourself. It makes you more present. On a physical level, it massages your internal organs and, with practice, your whole body.

Bobby: Someone once said to me, "When you learn how to breathe, you learn how to live." I began my training with breathing techniques by counting breaths—counting the inhalations and the exhalations—one for the inhale, two for the exhale, stopping at 10 and beginning again. For me this was difficult when I started. Somehow I would end up on 17 because my mind would wander so much. Next, I trained single breaths—one inhalation and one exhalation over the course of 1 minute and 30 seconds. For me, learning and practicing these breathing techniques has resulted in physical, mental and emotional strength as well as a clean alkalized body. I've also found that lengthening the inhalation increases my metabolism.

Mariel: Something I have learned through practicing yoga is that, by focusing, you can actually direct your breath into certain parts of your body—to heal them, to become more flexible, to become more conscious of that part, or even to become aware of an emotion stored there. Emotions get stored in the body, and they stay there until they are released. A powerful way of accessing, listening to and releasing a past trauma on your own is by directing the breath to the part of the body that stores that emotion or trauma. Breath unlocks that emotion or trauma and brings it into your awareness in the present moment, which is the only place it can actually be healed. Like I shared earlier, this type of focused breathing, combined with the intention of releasing a difficult memory, allowed me to transform my conditioned response to the smell of jasmine from negative to positive.

Stephen Elliott, author of *The New Science of Breath*, has developed a formal method of mindful breathing called Coherent Breathing. Elliott believes that imbalance of the autonomic nervous system may well be at the root of many current health issues such as anxiety and hypertension. Coherent Breathing promotes optimal respiration and blood flow and balances the breath cycle with the intrinsic autonomic nervous system rhythm and is highly effective in contributing to overall health, well-being and performance in daily life. A humanitarian group in southern Sudan called Goats for the Old Goat uses

Coherent Breathing with powerful results in helping to address post-traumatic stress disorder in individuals who are suffering the effects of war and slavery.

Breath and Being Present

Being present starts with each breath we take. We become more aware through our breath, and this is the first step to becoming conscious of our body and mind. Making this connection from the simple to the extreme by focusing on the breath in any everyday movement—from making tea or pouring a glass of water to training for an event—brings an awareness of our actions, and with that awareness, our movement becomes effortless. This is a form of meditation. Beginning meditators often start with the simple observation of breathing.

As you can see, it's not always about sitting. Sitting is a place to start—often people meditate in a seated position. But conscious awareness of your breath during your actions, whatever they are, can bring you to that meditative state.

A breath cannot happen over there—it cannot happen somewhere else. It is only happening right here, right now, within you. Breathing is an entry point for your connection with yourself. It is the practice of being present.

We like to think of each breath as a brand-new moment in our lives—and remember, we have 86,400 moments each day. Every inhale is the birth of a new moment, and every exhale is its release, a micro version of the life and death cycle. Each breath, each inhale and exhale, is another opportunity to consciously change and release the things that no longer serve us well and allow us to start anew.

You can create key times of your day—maybe sunrises or sunsets—to breathe in an intention with pointed focus and exhale a belief, thought, habit or experience that is negative or is working against you.

Breathing for Empowerment

We all have the power to become great! There are simple things that you can do to increase your awareness of how extraordinary you

already are. Inhale a huge amount of oxygen and imagine it traveling throughout your body and know that it is giving all of your cells
energy. Another way to create movement in your cells is to expel
short amounts of breath in rapid succession—this can totally re-
energize you if you're fatigued. Direct breath into areas of pain to
release the tension or the emotions causing it. Researchers have
found that patients who do breathing exercises before surgery are
less likely to suffer from pneumonia afterward (*pneuma,* by the way,
is Greek for "breath"). Breathing is powerful. It empowers you, and
it's free.

Many psychologists recommend breathing techniques for controlling our impulses and emotional reactions. If you're getting angry, for
example, doing some sort of breath work—whether it is a sudden,
short gasp through the throat or repeated slow, deep breaths through
the nose—will give you that moment of space needed to stop the
momentum of your anger. That window allows you to acknowledge
the feeling and make a new choice. Conscious breathing connects you
to your intuition or inner knowing, allowing you to respond with wisdom instead of being driven by the primitive part of your brain that
reacts with a fight-or-flight instinct.

On a spiritual level, by breathing deeply, you change your frequency. You actually shift how you are feeling through conscious
inhales and exhales. You become aware of the world from a different
perspective and become connected to the simplicity of what is happening right now rather than dwelling on stressful thoughts from
the past or contemplating the future. Conscious breathing accelerates
that process and brings you into the NOW. Just three or four deep,
conscious breaths will take you there. The late J. Krishnamurti, a
renowned writer and speaker on philosophical and spiritual subjects,
advised people who were going through a difficult period to take a
walk around the block while paying attention to their breath. While
this exercise obviously would not make a challenging situation disappear, Krishnamurti knew that even in the midst of difficulty, the
practice of deep breathing and moving has the power to change your
feelings, your thoughts, your consciousness and your energy level,
opening you up to the awareness of new options.

Breathing Exercises

Start by sitting quietly and comfortably on a chair or crossed-legged on the ground. First, take deep, measured breaths in and out through the nose. Nasal breathing stimulates the glands and heats up the body. To breathe more deeply, we suggest envisioning a vortex of light as it descends down into the top of your head into an opening that allows the light to enter and flood the body with energy. This visualization actually helps you focus and become conscious of your breath's power.

Below we describe some conscious breathing techniques. Start doing a little at a time and only as much as you feel comfortable with. If you feel lightheaded, stop and resume regular breathing.

Alternate Nostril Breathing

Alternate nostril breathing helps balance the right and left hemispheres of the brain. Called *nadi sodhana* in Sanskrit (that gives you an idea of how long it's been around), it helps you regain your equilibrium if you're feeling a little off. Here's how to do it:

Raise your right hand and place your right thumb on the right side of your nose. Bend your second and third fingers away from the nose, then place your pinky and ring finger on the left side of your nose. Close your *left* nostril by applying just enough pressure with your ring finger, and then inhale for a count of four through your *right* nostril. At the top of the inhale, hold your breath for a count of two.

Close your *right* nostril by pressing it with your thumb, and exhale through your *left* nostril (releasing your ring and pinky fingers). At the bottom of your exhale, hold your breath for a count of two.

Now repeat, inhaling on your *left* side and closing your *right* nostril with your thumb. Hold for a count of two. Exhale from your right nostril.

Inhale right, exhale left, inhale left, exhale right, inhale right, exhale left, etc. You'll always inhale on the side you just exhaled through. Go slowly and don't hyperventilate!

Start with five breaths on each side and see how you feel. A good rule of thumb is to hold your breath for a count that's half the count of your inhale. So if you inhale for four counts, hold for two. If you inhale for six counts, hold for three, and so on.

> *Bobby: Controlling the breath does not necessarily mean holding it. It's a question of focusing on the style of oxygenation you want. By taking deep breaths, you don't need as many. It's this kind of breathing that I usually do in the morning. I'll take one breath every minute or two, but my heart rate is exactly the same as it normally is. I'll do this for 10 to 15 breaths and get into a very relaxed state. This kind of exercise helps increase lung capacity and endurance.*

The Stimulating Breath (Bellows Breath)

The stimulating breath was adapted from a yoga breathing technique called *bhastrika*. (It has also been called a bellows breath after the device that forcefully blows air at a fire.) This exercise raises your energy level and makes you feel more alert. Here's how it works:

Inhale and exhale rapidly through your nose, keeping your mouth closed but relaxed. Your breaths in and out should be equal in duration, but as short as possible. This is a noisy breathing exercise.

Try for three in-and-out breath cycles per second. This produces a quick movement of the diaphragm, suggesting a bellows. Breathe normally after each cycle. Do not do this for more than 15 seconds on your first try. Each time you practice the stimulating breath, you can increase your time by five seconds or so until you reach a full minute.

If done properly, you may feel invigorated, comparable to the heightened awareness you feel after a good workout. You should feel the effort at the back of the neck, the diaphragm, the chest and the abdomen. Try this exercise anytime you feel that energy dip in the afternoon and think you need a candy bar or a cup of coffee. This is an amazing quick fix!

The Relaxing Breath

You can perform the relaxing breath exercise (also known as 4:7:8) when you want to calm and center yourself in silence. It's a great exercise to do when you've unplugged from technology and just want to connect with You. The relaxing breath exercise is so simple it can be done anywhere in any position, though we recommend that in the beginning as you are learning you sit with your back straight.

Place the tip of your tongue against the ridge of tissue just behind your upper front teeth, and keep it there through the entire exercise. You will be exhaling through your mouth around your tongue; try pursing your lips slightly if this seems awkward.

- Exhale completely through your mouth, making a whoosh sound. Close your mouth and inhale quietly through your nose to a mental count of four. Hold your breath for a count of seven.

- Exhale completely through your mouth, making a whoosh sound to a count of eight. This is one breath.

- Now inhale again and repeat the cycle three more times for a total of four breaths.

A few things to remember: always inhale quietly through your nose and exhale audibly through your mouth; the tip of your tongue stays in position behind your upper front teeth the whole time, and exhalation takes twice as long as inhalation. The absolute time you spend on each phase is not important; the ratio of 4:7:8 is what matters most. If you have trouble holding your breath, speed up the count but keep to the ratio of 4:7:8 for the three phases. With practice, you can slow it all down and get used to inhaling and exhaling more deeply.

This practice relaxes the nervous system. It's subtle at first but gains power with repetition. Try it at least twice a day. Don't do more than four rounds per session for the first month of practice. In time, you can build up to eight.

Breath Counting

Breath counting is a deceptively difficult practice, somewhat meditative, but very powerful. The more often you do this exercise, the stronger your lungs become and the more centered and focused you'll be in movement. Start practicing this while sitting, but you can later employ it while walking or hiking as well.

Sit in a comfortable position with your spine straight and your head inclined slightly forward. Gently close your eyes and take a few deep breaths. Then let the breath come naturally without trying to influence it. Ideally, it will be quiet and slow, but depth and rhythm may vary.

- To begin the exercise, count "one" to yourself as you exhale.

- The next time you exhale, count "two," and so on up to "five."

- Then begin a new cycle, counting "one" on the next exhalation.

Never count higher than "five," and count only when you exhale. You will know your attention has wandered when you find yourself up to "8," "12," even "19."

Try to do this exercise (which is also a form of meditation) for 10 minutes.

> *Mariel: I use breathing exercises with powerful results when I'm tired. Inhaling and holding the breath can actually bring energy to the body if you need a quick burst. A variation on this exercise is inhaling while tensing all your muscles and then releasing. This will bring energy to the whole body. These breathing exercises are so simple and they work!*

POINT-EARNING ACTIVITIES CHECKLIST

BREATHE CONSCIOUSLY

- Be mindful of your breath throughout the day. If you're in traffic or late for an appointment, check in with your breath. Focusing on your inhales and exhales releases your anxiety. **10 POINTS**

- Sit quietly and listen to your breath. Just observe. Inhale deeply. Exhale deeply. Observe what your diaphragm is doing. Are you breathing through your nose or your mouth? Try switching and see how that feels. That's it. (You'll be a step ahead for Chapter 4 when we talk about meditation!). **10 POINTS**

- Pick five moments in different parts of your day to breathe deeply into your lungs right into the base of your spine. **10 POINTS**

- Spend 15 minutes practicing any one of the four breathing exercises in this chapter. **10 POINTS**

- Breathe through your nose, especially while hiking, walking, biking or working out to oxygenate your muscles and organs and steady your mind. **10 POINTS**

- If you're feeling tightness or pain anywhere in your body, close your eyes and breathe into it. Visualize the spot and imagine oxygen surrounding and infiltrating the area. Exhale and see if you can release some tension in the process. Repeat this for ten breaths and see how you feel. **10 POINTS**

- If you find yourself in a blur of anger or frustration, step back and inhale deeply. Check in with your wiser self and reconsider your course of action. This one gets bonus points—it's not easy to stop the momentum of our temper, but the rewards are substantial. **20 POINTS**

- While lying in bed before going to sleep, notice how
  your breath changes. Then imagine a baby and mimic
  a baby's breath. Inhale, allowing your belly to puff up;
  exhale with a sigh of relief.   **5 POINTS**

- Squeeze your entire body—face, nose, eyes; simply
  squeeze *everything* on an inhale, hold two counts,
  and release on an exhale. See if you feel more
  focused or energetic.   **5 POINTS**

TOTAL POINTS _____

CHAPTER 4

LIVE SILENCE

Though silence is elusive, it is the key to fully experiencing and being present in your life. Silence exists between the sounds of everything going on around you—between the computer tapping, the music notes, the YouTube videos, the meetings, calls, cars, horns, blowers, mowers and airplanes that fill our world with noise. When we learn to embrace the silence, to even make space for prolonged periods of silence, we find that we are powerful beyond belief. Silence is the space, the energy, from which we can create and re-create our reality.

It is rare to experience true silence but important to commit to it. Stilling your brain through listening to nothing more than the sounds of Nature or your breath is a commitment to figuring yourself out. Take moments before or during your morning ritual (or anytime you can grab a moment away from NOISE) where you sit in stillness and all you hear is your breath. Relinquish the need to do anything in this place. For while doing nothing, everything is happening. The Buddhist monks say, "Nothingness is the Isness."

It is in silence where your inner voice can be heard. Create silent space for yourself, where you can develop a relationship with that voice and unlock the door to the truth of you. If you can make quiet time part of your daily routine, you will be among those who truly know themselves and are able to see themselves, be themselves and be a part of what is actually taking place in the world around them. When there is silence, truth makes itself known to you.

> *Mariel: Connection begins in silence. Connection is what you feel when you are completely present with yourself, when everything else seems to disappear and you are aware of only what you feel inside. Connection happens with Self first, so silence is how you ignite a connection with you. Silence shines light on how you are feeling in your inner world. When we are connected with our inner world, we are able to connect in a healthier way with our outer world—with deeper understanding of ourselves, our actions and the role we play.*

> *Bobby: If you can't live inside yourself, where are you going to live? Outside yourself, always needing someone or something. Need nothing; be part of everything; and work with what you have.*

Intuition (Inner Knowing)

In silent stillness (assuming you aren't over-caffeinated, over-chemicalized, over-sugared or under-slept), you have an openness about you. Information settles in more easily, and you can later apply it in far more productive and effective ways. If you get rid of the noise, you can actually *hear yourself*—hear your thoughts, hear your needs, hear that inner voice that is your intuition.

You may receive an instruction or a piece of information that sounds different from your usual thoughts while practicing silence. The thought may have a different resonance—it sounds like you and yet it doesn't, as though it's a message from a more balanced version of yourself. This is your own wisdom coming to you . . . this is your intuition, or inner knowing. This is YOU clear and uncomplicated, ready to guide your every move. Listen and trust in what you hear. The more you are in silence, the more valuable information for your life you will receive. Initially, you may feel unsure about what you feel or hear, but with time you will grow confident that the messenger inside is YOU—your greatest champion.

Mariel: Silence is the key to growth. Bobby and I take silent moments, alone, every day. Whether in Nature, in the yard or before getting out of bed in the morning, we take time to listen to what is going on in our inner world. If you don't get silent, how can you hear what is going on inside of you? We can so easily run around "doing" our lives making this and that thing, person or appointment more important than our inner voice. By going quiet, we can tune into ourselves.

In silence lives patience, happiness and self-acceptance. Always remember, we are never separate from this place. When we understand this, we are in our truth. Who we actually are, who we were and who we can become is always within us and around us. Sometimes we have to remind ourselves of this. In this profound silence, we will find the answers.

Meditation: Tuning Out to Tune In

Meditation is a way to distill and maximize periods of silence. This centuries-old practice helps bring focus, not only in the quiet intervals, but in all other parts of your life as well. Scientists know and verify what meditation does to the brain and how it improves mental, emotional and physical health. Studies have suggested that it can boost the immune system, lower the perception of pain, decrease anxiety, cure insomnia and inhibit the production of cortisol, a stress hormone. One study found that subjects who meditated for 20 minutes a day were less sensitive to pain after only three days!

Scientists have found that meditation has a physical effect on the brain; it thickens the cerebral cortex. In one well-known study at the University of Washington, brain maps of Tibetan monks who were experienced meditators (some with more than 10,000 hours of silent sitting) showed remarkably strong gamma-wave activity while the monks meditated on the idea of compassion. Gamma waves, believed to be responsible for our perception of consciousness, are usually extremely hard to detect. But the gamma waves exhibited by the meditating monks weren't just powerful, they were coordinated between different areas of the cortex, as they would be if someone were under anesthesia. The left prefrontal cortex of the monks' brains, the area of happiness and positive emotions, was especially active during their meditation. These particular monks were students of the Dalai Lama, who has a longstanding interest in exploring the science of meditation.

Another study found that Transcendental Meditation (TM—a specific form of meditation) helped patients with coronary heart disease prevent subsequent heart attacks and strokes. And researchers at the University of Oregon discovered that meditation can help stave off memory loss, a finding that may be developed further to help the growing population of people with Alzheimer's disease.

Meditation Made Easy

Meditation requires you only to show up and get quiet. This can be done anywhere, any place, any time. It can be done in stillness and in movement. The movement can be anything—writing, painting, dancing, running, walking. It can happen during athletic movement or an event and, of course, while laughing and playing. It's the commitment of being fully connected anywhere. People connect to silence in many ways, and finding stillness during activity is an amazing experience worth working on.

You can create a special area. You can stand, sit, kneel or even lay down—whatever helps you to connect, relax and tune in. Whether moving or sitting still, you still connect to the same pure place, and the experience of who you are reveals itself. The more you connect, the more powerful you become. When not moving, you can engage in meditation with eyes open or closed. With your eyes open, you can focus on what is in front of you whether it is a flower, the flame of a candle, a tree, a mountain, the clouds, your breath on a cold day or even ants crawling on the ground. Silence is profound, and it is in and around everything. The goal is to still your mind. Any kind of action that you do quietly with internal stillness is a meditation—the monks find stillness and meditation in everything they do—listening, smiling, making a bed, chopping wood, gardening, painting a picture, walking in Nature.

Mariel: When I first started meditating, I did it for only five minutes at a time. Then every couple of days I added one more minute until eventually I was up to 20 then 30 minutes twice a day. While I find that this really works for me, it may be too much for others. It's about finding what length of time is right for you. Start with five minutes like I did and see where it goes from there.

Initially, sitting alone with yourself may feel uncomfortable. Start slowly. Even two to five minutes is a good beginning. You'll find that you'll be able to be quiet in many places—and in time, with or without other people around you. You will notice that silence is everywhere. You can enjoy moments of silence anywhere from the beach to the bus stop, from waiting in line to going for a walk. Take the time when it is given to you. Observe your inhales and your exhales. Breathing is always a way to check in with yourself. Listen to your thoughts; do you feel angry, happy, sad, hungry, thirsty or bored? And then ask yourself, "Who am I being right now? Is this my choice?" Make a conscious choice to be what and who you want to be in this moment.

Be curious about quietness. See how loud it can be—the buzz of a bee or a fly, a hum from the electronics in the room. Notice these sounds, but don't hold onto them. They are the white noise—the backdrop for the sound of your inner voice.

Allow yourself to have every thought and feeling as you meditate, making nothing bad or wrong. Though we may find some thoughts shameful, judgmental or embarrassing, this is merely a reaction of the unconscious mind. For instance, as you begin to quiet yourself for meditation, you might think to yourself, "There is no time for this. . . ." Guilt has no place in your silent time. Simply observe that thought—don't give it a negative or a positive charge. It has no power in this moment. Let it pass.

The idea is to be the objective observer of what surfaces in your mind. Oftentimes these thoughts are unconscious and reactive to what someone else has told us and not at all what is actually taking place now. Make it your goal to see things for what they are rather than what you think they are. Remind yourself that you will always have thoughts; it is what you do with them when they come up that matters. Allow them and let them go. When you do this, you might have an epiphany or "aha" moment that you are not your thoughts. This is profound.

As Miguel Ruiz teaches in *The Fifth Agreement: A Practical Guide to Self-Mastery,* when we believe false ideas, they pull us away from our authentic Self. In meditation, we can let go of the power these ideas have had on our lives. We can allow our feelings and thoughts to rise without judgment and watch them go.

It is our practice not to buy into feelings that cause anxiety or pain. We are fine for feeling them, and we are even happier (if not healthier) for letting them go. We can choose to handle them in a constructive way. When we accept our feelings as natural, normal, healthy and productive ways of communicating with our inner Self, we are much less likely to act out on them inappropriately in ways that hurt ourselves or others.

Acknowledging and accepting our feelings leads to acceptance of our entire being. When we are aware of how we show up in our lives day to day, we are more able to have healthy, productive relationships. How can we understand and have compassion for others when we can't understand or care for ourselves? Our relationship with our Self is the most important one we have.

Prayer

Prayer and meditation are subtle in their difference, and both may be practiced during a period of quiet contemplation, or "sitting" as it is sometimes called. In meditation, we receive information from our inner Self, from the Universe, from God or our higher power. In prayer, we ask one or all of those entities for help. We put it out there: "I really need help figuring out what this means." When we ask for understanding, we are asking the deepest part of our being for clarity. Answers come from within us. That is why the connection of meditation with prayer is powerful—because the stillness achieved in meditation allows us to connect powerfully to our inner voice, and when we make that connection we have space for guidance to be received. Sometimes answers arrive at strange times. You may "figure it out" standing in line at the grocery store or while riding your bike. A "drop in" can happen at any moment, and when it comes, you feel a sense of peace knowing your answer is there.

When this sort of thing happens, you begin to realize the synchronicity of life, the perfect timing that goes beyond coincidence. Perhaps it's hearing the same information told in a slightly different way from three different sources in the same vicinity of time. You start to realize that when you pay attention, the information comes your way. Being aware of this allows you to act on it.

Meditation, stillness and silence can all help you recognize the messages as they come across your path. You can develop an acute ability to hear your intuition, your authority, your instinctive power to heal. Our inner resources are vast and powerful, but we can only access them by listening. Poor lifestyle choices like lack of sleep or overindulgence can inhibit our ability to listen. *Running with Nature* is about inspiring you toward healthy lifestyle choices that create an environment for conscious listening.

> *Mariel: My inner voice speaks to me in my own way. Bobby's inner voice speaks to him in his own way. If we never got silent, we'd never hear them. The types of food that we eat and the exercises we do, all our lifestyle choices, help us to feel the resonance of silence, to experience ourselves as we really are. You can't feel yourself within noise, distraction and environmental inundation. And since we are so used to noise, you may find it uncomfortable at first to sit in silence. Try not to turn on the TV for background noise when you come home from work, or try driving without the radio on. It may feel like awkward silence; just acknowledge that feeling and see how long you can continue in silence. Find other things in your life that you can do without distracting sound. It's so worth it.*

One more note about prayer that we find valuable—when asking God or the Universe or whatever supreme being you believe in for something, whether it is a job or to be out of pain or for the well-being of someone you love, always add this phrase in your head, "For the highest good of all concerned in connection to the universe and the source of all that is." We can't always see the big picture in a given circumstance. We don't always see what's best from our perspective. Our idea is for greater peace and happiness for ourselves or for others, and what we truly want is what will get us there, not just what we *think* will get us there.

> *Bobby: My meditation practice is all about the breath—long, deep breaths in and long deep breaths out, until I get into a pattern. It's a very simple inhale and exhale. I listen to my breath. If you put earplugs in or headphones on, you can amplify the sound of your breath. It's that Darth Vader kind of breathing that comes from the back of your throat. I always inhale through my nose and exhale out through my mouth.*

Universal Energy

We believe that the world is run by a higher energy source that is beyond seeing, touching, hearing, smelling and tasting. It is an intelligent energy with a much larger understanding of the big picture than we are all connected to. This may sound like a contradiction of what we've been saying about being your own authority, but it isn't. This intelligent energy, we believe, is responsible for creating us and everything else in the world, and we have access to it through our authentic Self. We hold the intelligence of this higher power, or higher energy, within our own being. Thus we are part of it. We believe that when you get attuned to your authentic Self, you are able to access your own uniqueness and path in life. You find that your greatest teacher is within.

Hearing Ourselves

In silence, in meditation and in prayer, thoughts and feelings and memories will come up. When we finally quiet the distractions of the mind, what's lurking beneath the surface reveals itself. Like everything else in Nature, we are designed to heal and expand. The unresolved thoughts, feelings and memories surface to be addressed. And while revisiting them may be the last thing we want to do, it may be the very best thing to do. They may lead us to a deeper understanding of ourselves and answer questions that bring us to a place of wholeness and well-being.

In the case of severe trauma or depression, it's best to work with a qualified counselor or teacher during this process. You may need the assurance that whatever memories present themselves, you are in a safe place to deal with them. This counselor or teacher can provide you with an opening to resolve your past and enable you to move forward. When a person continues to hold onto bad memories, they create all kinds of distractions for themselves. Those memories have a way of revealing themselves in a negative way. Their toxic buildup will eventually release itself through volatile emotions, unhealthy habits, physical disease and automatic reactions rather than responses.

We have found that memories—as upsetting or frightening as they may have once been—appear in meditation like pictures on a screen. They come up, we look at them, we see how they make us feel, and then they leave. Though the feelings may be intense at times, the charge or emotional intensity diminishes each time they're permitted to pass through the body without comment and be released. Always remember that memories are just memories—they cannot hurt you any longer. It's a tremendous relief to be able to address feelings that come up from our past, because likely we were unable or not allowed to address them as a child.

In many families, certain feelings are okay, but others are not. It's acceptable to feel happy but never sad. You can feel mildly frustrated but never angry. It is fine to feel ashamed, but you can never feel proud of yourself. In meditation, it is common to get in touch with these feelings for the first time. Sometimes just allowing yourself to have these feelings releases them.

Truth simply cannot be denied forever. More important, the truth, even if it is momentarily painful, has an amazing power to heal. Acknowledging and releasing pent-up emotions is another form of cleansing—emotional cleansing. When we refuse to acknowledge or really feel our feelings, they manifest as poor health. When we suppress an emotion, the energy of that emotion does not go away. It simply sinks deeper into the physical body.

As scientists of mind-body medicine have known for decades, our emotional toxicity causes physical disease. By bringing awareness to these feelings, you strip them of their power. This leaves you better able to move forward emotionally and physically. It gets you unstuck.

Meditation is a wonderful opportunity to look at the inner Self and to discover what lies hidden inside YOU. When we acknowledge our upsets, our anger and our fears, these "e-motions"—energies that are in motion—dissipate. Denying their existence only strengthens their hold.

What's truly exciting about silence is that you can treat it as a project. Instead of saying to yourself, "I'm scared of what's coming," say to yourself, "I'm excited to learn about me; I am a scientist on a journey of my own self discovery." Then whatever comes up becomes an interesting clue to YOU and why you behave the way you do.

A Higher Level of Conscious Living

Science is beginning to agree with the Law of Attraction—the concept that like matter attracts like matter. If we are negative and angry, other negative and angry people seem to show up in our lives. Likewise, if we're happy, we seem to attract other happy people. If we're intelligent, we generally have intelligent friends. So as you become more aware, you may find yourself shifting toward having more aware people in your life.

By sitting in silence and observing your thoughts each day, you will start exercising your power of choice in more areas of your life. Taking time for silence will bring you to a higher level of conscious living overall. Mindfulness will be incorporated into everything you do. As a result, you will be living more in accordance with your own truth—stepping into a life that is true for you.

Everything we are sharing with you is about waking up to the truth of YOU, and silence is one of the most important habits you will acquire on your path to living your best life.

Bobby: There's a constant bombardment of information and noise in our society. As a result, many people think they need external input to function. That mindset abdicates the authority over their lives to forces outside themselves. We really don't need an outside authority to tell us how to be. The path of truth is different for each of us. No one else can tell you what is true for you. When you become quiet and get beyond the discomfort of losing that outside input, you start to know—I'm talking about an overall knowing, a wisdom. The moment you stop listening to your own inner voice and begin following someone else, you cease following your own truth.

Turn OFF Technology

Even when our e-devices are not making a lot of sound, they still create a noisy environment, bombarding us with information, some useful, some mindless and distracting. This is why we highly recommend that you take at least one entire day off a week from technology. And find time each day, even if only for a few moments, that is as technology free as possible.

If the first thing you do in the morning is turn on your computer and check email—and trust us, we have done this as well—it sets you up for a different kind of day energetically than if you begin by moving slowly and consciously, with a mindful ritual in a space that honors you. Email alone can become demanding when you answer every message in your inbox. It's interesting how we give other people an open invitation into our lives 24/7 through technology—tweets, texts, phone calls, emails—we are constantly "on call." When technology rules, it creates a seemingly endless string of tasks to complete. When we give ourselves quiet space, we gain perspective on what is important; we use our imaginations to create our day—this is far more powerful than any computer.

Mariel: During my meditation, at first I concentrate on deep nasal breathing. I visualize my breath rising up through my spine on my inhales and down my spine and into the center of the earth on my exhales. I see my breath as light traveling up my spine through the top of my head to the farthest star I can imagine and down again through to the core of the earth.

Once my breath has filled me with a deep calm inside, my meditation really becomes about being aware of all my senses. I focus on every sensation around me—a breeze, dampness, smells, sound. When you become silent, you realize there is so much sound, and with attentiveness, you can distinguish and hear each one separately.

Starting Your Practice of Meditation

Here are a few ideas on how to start your own meditation practice.

Set Aside Time

Mornings and evenings are good times for meditation. Monks often rise at 4 a.m. for their first sitting, a time when the rest of the world is asleep and the earth's energy has yet to be distracted by humans. While this might be too early for the rest of us, a meditation before breakfast is an awesome way to start the day. An early evening meditation while watching the sunset is a peaceful way to enter that time when the energy of the day begins to wind down, when work is done and we begin to settle into the evening.

Carving out even five minutes for silence and/or meditation can dramatically affect your state of mind. Gradually you can extend the duration, maybe to 20 minutes twice a day or longer. Meditation expands time. By making time for YOU, you calm the frenetic pace of your life. Taking time for regular meditation makes your days flow with ease and makes you present.

Think back to when you were say, twelve years old, and you walked or rode your bike everywhere. When you got of school in June, your thoughts were, "Wow, no school until next year!" Summer seemed to last forever, and actually it was only 12 weeks. We were at an age when we lived each moment, and because of this, the days seemed longer . . . summer felt like a year. If you were to give most adults a deadline of 12 weeks for a major project, they would say that is not enough time. The number of hours is the same, but the perspective is different. With age everything seems to speed up. We say things like, "I can't believe it's Christmas again" or "I can't believe summer is already over." Another birthday, another anniversary, another milestone seems to have come and gone so quickly. How we see things brings the illusion of time moving faster or slower. Meditation brings us back to the present moment like when we were young. This is one of the most valuable assets . . . real time . . . the present moment. It enables us to see things for how they are instead of how we think they are.

Find a Space

Create a space in a quiet part of your home or in Nature. When we create this quiet space, it becomes part of us; we awaken the silence within ourselves and it goes with us everywhere. Like we mentioned before, silence and meditation can also be found while moving. Moving meditation is powerful, finding the stillness within even while our bodies are engaged in activity. This is where athletes and artists are at their best. There is a sense of freedom that anything is possible. This is called many things—*being in the moment, the zone* or *satori*. Finding quiet in all parts of your life is key to true connection to yourself and your higher consciousness.

While practicing sitting meditation, we prefer sitting on the floor or on a cushion or when outside on the ground or a blanket, but you may be more comfortable in a chair or on a pillow with your back supported by a wall. The important thing is that you're comfortable. Lying down is an option, but beginners are often inclined to go to sleep if they get too comfy.

For you moms out there who have little ones, take your silent time while they nap or while you rock your baby to sleep.

Empty Your Stomach

It's okay to have a cup of tea before you meditate, but we recommend doing it on an otherwise empty stomach. Your mind is clearer when your body isn't busy digesting, and you'll get much more out of your practice.

Begin with Breath

When you've settled into your meditation space, take a few deep breaths and think about any intentions you might have. Do you want to devote this practice to a person or perhaps to a cause? Let's say you intend to devote your meditation to world peace. Envision personal "peace" on the inhale. As you exhale, imagine your sense of peace and that same peace enveloping the world around you. You are sending positive energy toward your cause. This can be done with any focus.

Do this for four or five unhurried inhales and equally unhurried exhales. Ideally, your inhale and exhale will be the same length. Now let the intention go. Be still and listen.

If thoughts or outside sounds arise, allow them in and let them out. You might want to imagine you have two doors in your mind, both of them wide open. Thoughts and sounds breeze in through one door and out through the other, disturbing nothing on their route. They are inconsequential elements of the present moment, and you are the present moment's observer. Notice without drawing conclusions or judging your thoughts.

That's all there is to it! If you find your thoughts taking over—which they likely will—just go back to focusing on your breath. Start simply by counting your breaths—one, inhale; two, exhale; three, inhale; four, exhale; and so on. Each breath is long and deep matched by a long and deep exhale of the same length. Start by counting to ten and start over again. With practice, you'll notice you won't have to count anymore; you'll begin to naturally follow your breaths.

When you begin to let go of conscious thought, your intuitive mind will take over the meditation. Listen and watch. Once you're in tune, your intuitive mind will also tell you when your session is up. It will turn out to be the perfect amount of time for you.

Soon you find a peacefulness spreading throughout your body, then you make the connection with your mind, and finally you begin to understand this elusive word we call Spirit. Make this practice part of your day, and that same peacefulness will be infused into the rest of your life.

Walking Meditation

A walking meditation combines movement and mindfulness. You can do a walking meditation in your neighborhood, in the mountains or on the beach—anywhere you can move freely and let your thoughts come and go.

During a walking meditation, you watch, listen, smell and become hyperaware of your environment. You may want to touch the leaves, let sand fall through your fingers or stop to watch a bird fly. Whatever is going on in the moment, allow yourself to experience it, take it in. Feel your body in motion and become acquainted with how you truly feel. Don't run from any sensation or breath. Watch how you observe the world. Are you bothered by noise or easily distracted? No big deal. Just let yourself feel it.

As with any meditation, a walking meditation is about getting in touch with You. We believe stillness in motion is an art form. Observe yourself without judgment. See how you fit into the landscape. The more you meditate, whether in motion or in stillness, the more finely you will adjust the balance of your body, mind and spirit.

POINT-EARNING ACTIVITIES CHECKLIST

LIVE SILENCE

- Sit silently for 10 minutes before breakfast in the morning.   **10 POINTS**

- Go outside for a 20-minute walking meditation in the morning.   **10 POINTS**

- Three times throughout the day, stop what you are doing, find a quiet place, shut your eyes and empty your mind. Breathe mindfully.   **10 POINTS**

- Create a sacred space that reflects You.   **10 POINTS**

- While you are going about a daily routine—cooking, making lunch, dressing—see if you can do it with quiet mindfulness. Feel the buttons on your shirt as they go through the buttonholes, the insole of your shoe against the arch of your foot, the comb going through your hair. Awareness can make the mundane amazing.   **10 POINTS**

- Sit and watch a sunset and meditate as the sun goes down. Let go of the stress of your day.   **10 POINTS**

- Meditate for 10 to 20 minutes in the morning and the evening for one week without interruption. Follow the meditation tips in the chapter. Record how you feel after the first meditation and after the last.   **10 POINTS**

- During your drive time or commute time this week, try to take the first 10 minutes to practice being aware by becoming an objective, non-judgmental observer of everything around you.   **5 POINTS**

- Do an Internet search on "meditation in everyday life" and see how others incorporate meditation into their daily routines. Do not make this an extensive research project. It's just about learning something helpful for your everyday practice.   **5 POINTS**

- Try going technology-free for the first hour and last two hours of the day—no phone calls, emails or computer time. Notice any feelings that emerge and any patterns that you become of aware of.   **10 POINTS**

TOTAL POINTS _____

CHAPTER 5

EAT WHOLESOME FOOD

There is more controversy about food than almost any other subject on the planet. Nearly every question you can imagine has been asked and explored on the topic—what, where, when, how and why we eat. We hope to give you some insight into the labyrinth of the food world and inspire you to discover your individual needs. We have been here over 8,000 years, flown men to the moon, and still can't figure out how to eat. We believe that just as the seasons change, so do our day-to-day lives. Some days or weeks we go nonstop—whether it's athletics, our jobs or chasing our kids around in all directions. Other days are slower and more relaxed. We must learn to make adjustments with our food to mirror what's happening in our lives— more activity means more calories for energy; a slower pace means we don't eat as much, or at least not as many calories. There is no one-size-fits-all guidebook on how to eat. There are many diverse cultures, climates and seasons to consider, not to mention body types, metabolisms and genetics.

Some experts believe blood types are a factor as well. Mariel is type A, which means she leans toward mostly greens and vegetables with lighter protein, nuts and seeds . . . maybe a little bit of a *granola girl* with a hint of *Tribeca* mixed in. Bobby, on the other hand, is type O, meaning he's okay with just about everything. He often says he can eat a pair of shoes and digest them. He leans toward raw meat and raw animal fat as well as greens, grains, fruits and vegetables . . .

perhaps we just call him a *GUY*. But for both of us, it is a balance that we figure out for ourselves every day.

Our heritage plays a role in the types of food we eat as well. Mariel is mostly English, along with a little Scottish and American Indian. Bobby is Scottish, Irish, English, Welsh and American Indian, plus on his mother's side there is Ukrainian, Lithuanian, Russian and Czech. We are all a mix of many cultures, habits and traditions. Many generations make up your unique genetic code, and all of that needs to be considered as you explore and establish your optimum food lifestyle. For instance, living in sub-zero temperatures where their livelihood is hunting and fishing, the Eskimos or Inuit eat a high fat, high protein (predominantly meat and 50 to 75 percent fat) diet because it supports their lifestyle. In India, where the temperatures are hot and 50 percent of the population grows and sells fruit and vegetables, they have the highest population of vegetarians—almost 40 percent. And those that do eat meat eat it infrequently.

With that in mind, we're going to share simple ideas and choices *we* make that will inspire you to find your own personal food system that will support you in being healthy, vibrant and strong for many years to come. Food is energy. You know the expression, "You are what you eat." Or maybe you've heard, "Live food, live body." The healthier and more vibrant the food we eat, the healthier we become.

Our bodies are constantly regenerating new blood, tissue, muscles, tendons, ligaments and bones. According to the Stanford School of Medicine, every cell in our skeleton is replaced every seven years. So what we put into our bodies determines how efficiently this regeneration process takes place. This is where the term "growing younger" comes from. Studies have shown that cells regenerate most effectively in a healthy environment with proper nutrition, whereas cells in an unhealthy environment degenerate—become weak and distorted. This is part of an accelerated aging process. Our experience is that we can slow down or even reverse this damage by the food we eat, the environment we live in and the lifestyle we choose.

When we eat food, a kind of partnership takes place . . . it is a transfer of energy from one place to another. For example, when you eat an apple, the life force of that apple continues on a journey with you. If the apple would have fallen to the ground and been left, that apple would go back into the earth and become part of the soil where it begins to grow again. When we pick the apple and eat it, the life force and energy moves forward with us. This is where an agreement is made between you and the apple. All of the information that came from the earth, the sun, the water, the soil and the seasons is inside the apple and then inside us.

This is similar to the Native Americans asking *the medicine* to accept them in order to heal. This is why we say a simple prayer before we eat, being thankful for the food, and all the hard work that has taken place prior to bringing it from *farm to table*. This is why it is so important to know where your food comes from and how it comes to you—organic, pesticide or spray-free, biodynamic or sustainable. The quality of your food equals the quality of your life. It's true . . . you really are what you eat.

Built for Longevity

We often start the day with a green juice—celery, parsley and spinach. A lot of times, we will turn it into a green power shake by adding up to 15 ingredients in our Vitamix Blender (see recipe on page 92). We feel this has a plethora of healing benefits: alkalizes the body, provides super-food nutrition and raises the frequency of your entire body, mind and spirit. And believe it or not, it tastes fantastic!

> *Bobby: Have you ever taken margarine out of the refrigerator and put it outside? Nothing will go near it. No flies, no bugs—nothing. Not an organism on the planet will live on it, not even mold. It doesn't matter how long you leave it out, it remains the same and eventually hardens up to have a plastic-like texture. Who wants to eat that?*

Obesity Is Not Inevitable

One of the reasons many Americans are overweight is because their friends and family are overweight. If all a person sees in their environment are heavy people, it begins to be accepted as the norm. The unbelievable part about this epidemic is that it is completely preventable. Obesity is rampant, especially in America, because people are not eating real food. Processed, drive-through fast food; deep-fried, sugar-filled, hormone-injected, factory-farmed meats; and high fructose corn syrup (HFCS) are making people fat, sick and unhappy. The diet soda accompanying the meal doesn't help matters—artificial sweeteners create an unnatural craving for more sugary-tasting foods that actually make you gain weight.

We are paying the price for our addiction to processed food. Think "addiction" is too strong a word? Studies have shown that fatty and sugary foods can hijack the brain in ways that resemble addictions to cocaine, nicotine and other drugs. So trying to change eating habits proves to be extremely challenging for many people. Here is the deal: You must make healthy food choices if you want to avoid obesity, diabetes, heart and lung disease and even some types of cancer. When you make a decision to change the way you eat, remember that it takes 21 days for an addictive pattern to be released from your brain. Twenty-one days to a new way of living is not that long in the scheme of things.

The advertising industry exerts an enormous amount of influence on our culture and especially on our children. They watch hours of television and are bombarded with unhealthful food ads for products that appear to make them happier, more popular and more like that sports star or celebrity they look up to. Kids beg for the foods they see on TV, and many parents succumb to the pressure. Hence childhood obesity is out of control. Wherever we go we are encouraged to eat junk food. Airports, billboards, the mall, the Internet—everywhere the message is: Eat poorly and be happy. It makes us sad.

The good news is that children and adults don't become overweight or obese from eating too many fruits and vegetables or protein and good fat in its pure form. By filling up on the fiber, vitamins and minerals that are plentiful in these foods, you can stave off cravings for the processed and unhealthy foods.

Start paying attention to the source and substance of what's in your grocery bags—the result will be a healthy and happier you.

Farmers Markets

There are some products you just can't find locally, but given the choice between a food that's been farmed within a hundred miles and one that's been flown in from another country, we'll always go local to minimize our carbon footprint. No one with any sense of environmental awareness wants to add to the world's toxic emissions by supporting a consumer market for foods flown across continents and shipped across seas.

That's why we're regulars at the local farmers markets—for the most part they're our grocery stores. We go to the best markets in our area, and sometimes we take a road trip to the ones outside our neighborhood. Not only is the food seasonal and straight from the farms, we can talk to the people who grow it and give them a fair price that's not stepped on by a distributor/middleman. In exchange, we know we're getting fresh local produce from small organic farms— no waxes, chemicals, sprays or colorings. Aside from fruits and vegetables, we also buy raw olive oils, nuts and cheeses, meat and poultry. The farmers, whose property has often been in the family for generations, put their lives and love into cultivating their produce and livestock, and you can taste it. By supporting them, you're supporting your health and the local economy. It's a win-win!

Seventy-five percent of Americans are within five miles of a local farmers market and don't know it. Look online for the closest local farmers market in your area and make it a habit to go once a week. It's easier than you think, and it's fun. It becomes part of your food's journey (remember our apple :)). You will enjoy food that you have carefully picked and prepared far more than you realize. While you're there, try a new organic food. Try a squash blossom in a stir-fry, snack on an Asian pear, or experience a rich, raw olive oil over heirloom tomatoes.

Mariel: Going to the farmers market for me has become a ritual I love. I stop and chat with farmers I have come to know, and they recommend the best of their crop. I love the colors of all the seasonal produce. I can't wait to buy from the sprout girl who sprouts just about everything: lentils, sunflower seeds, spicy radishes, onions, peas and broccoli to name a few. My mouth waters thinking of the salad recipe I will create after I buy local walnut oil that I'll use for a dressing. The whole experience becomes one of connection and community, and it feels good!

Keep It Simple

We eat a lot of raw food but not completely raw. Our philosophy is: buy the best ingredients you can find seasonally and do as little to them as possible. The idea is to enhance, rather than smother, the ingredients you've been so conscientious in sourcing. Blanching, steaming, sautéing and quickly searing vegetables, meats and fish is key to maximizing taste and nutrition. Some vegetables are healthier when cooked just a little bit. For instance, when broccoli is lightly steamed, the protective layer of skin is broken and allows the nutrients of the broccoli to be better absorbed.

When we're cooking at home, we like to keep it simple. Herbs, spices and good oils are the best ingredients for making *clean* food. Become accustomed to food in its most natural state. Once you start, you won't go back. Your sauces become various types of oils flavored with olives, garlic, onions, peppers and seasonings, fresh salsas and pesto. All of them are simple, nutritious and tasty. When you buy the best ingredients, you get the best flavor. When you buy a piece of fresh fish and you sauté or broil it with fresh herbs, *real salt* and pepper, and then a dash of olive oil, you can't find anything more delicious. The key to good food is how you cook it, not what you put over it to cover it up. With all their nutrients intact, not cooked out or compromised by excessive manipulation, these foods will do what they're programmed to do—keep you and your immune system healthy.

Chef and food activist Alice Waters, the founder of Chez Panisse—the 40-year-old restaurant in Berkeley, California, that sparked a revolution in American cooking—is a master of the less-is-more style. Waters and her cookbooks, including *The Art of Simple Food,* emphasize the rewards of keeping preparations simple.

Waters knows that the key to achieving healthy, delicious meals from the simplest preparation is to start with wholesome, fresh food. So for decades she has enlisted farmers to grow produce expressly for her restaurant, establishing a farm-to-table relationship that's become common for high-end chefs. She has taken this important concept a step further and is now working to ensure the health and welfare of future generations by raising money to fund food curriculums and gardens in schools through her Edible Schoolyard Project.

We need to teach kids about the powerful connection between food and health. By learning how to make healthy eating a natural part of everyday life, this generation will influence their children and generations to come. The cycle of indulging in processed, sugary, preservative-filled, nutrition-free foods has to end, and hands-on education is the most effective way to make that happen.

Toss Your Microwave!

This may sound ridiculous to some. It seems smart to cut 20 or 30 minutes off cooking time in order to give ourselves time for more valuable endeavors. But there is a huge price that we pay for this convenience. We threw our microwave out after learning that at one point they had been banned in Germany and Russia due to evidence that microwaved foods pose definite health threats. How? Food cooked in a microwave undergoes molecular changes that reduce its nutrient content and, in our view, make it a non-food. Not to mention it diminishes flavor.

Authors Mira Calton, CN, and Jayson Calton, Ph.D., discuss the nutritional effects of microwave cooking in their book *Naked Calories*. They cite a study done in Spain in which researchers measured the level of flavonoids (a type of health-producing antioxidant) that remained in broccoli after it was cooked by four popular cooking methods—steaming, pressure-cooking, boiling and microwaving. When compared with raw, fresh broccoli, steaming the broccoli had minimal effects in terms of loss; boiling led to a 66 percent loss of flavonoids; high pressure-cooking caused a 47 percent loss; and microwaving proved catastrophic with an almost complete elimination of 97 percent of the health-supporting flavonoids.

However, these molecular changes do more than just zap food of its optimum flavor and nutritional value. They affect the basic structure of the food in a way that, according to some studies, renders it carcinogenic. The conversation is (as you can imagine) controversial, and the language can get technical. If you feel the need to hold onto your fast-heating machine, we suggest you research it too and decide for yourself. One study to start with is that conducted by Dr. Hans Ulrich Hertel and Dr. Bernard H. Blanc of the Swiss Federal Institute of Technology and the University Institute for Biochemistry.

Practically speaking, a microwave is never going to sear your steak with a dark char on the outside and a red center, and it's not going to give you a hot baked potato with a dry crackly skin and feathery light interior. So if you own a microwave, go ahead and use it—as a big clock or a high-tech breadbox.

Eating Seasonally

Part of living in harmony with our true nature is living according to the rhythms of our natural environment. This includes eating seasonally—which you'll be doing if you buy most of your produce at farmers markets. Seasonal food gives our bodies what they need. Depending on the climate you live in, this may mean having warm or "snow foods" in the winter and more raw, cool "sun foods" in the summer. Examples of snow foods are kale, broccoli, root vegetables (carrots, turnips, parsnips, rutabagas), squashes, sweet potatoes and onions. Sun foods include corn, asparagus, artichokes, berries, papayas, peppers, lettuces, strawberries, peaches, blueberries and melons.

We enhance our base of fresh fruits and vegetables with lean and humanely raised meats and poultry, eggs, fresh fish and unpasteurized dairy. We never eat anything that is processed. We get fresh, raw milk (natural, unpasteurized) from a local dairy, and we order bison, which is an especially clean meat, from North Star Bison when we can't find it locally.

Achieving an Acid Alkaline Balance

You probably remember doing experiments with pH strips in high school science class. The strips determine whether a solution is acidic, with a pH of 1 to 7, or alkaline, with a pH of 7 to 14. The body, too, can be acid or alkaline, but ideally it falls right in the middle, with a pH between 7.35 and 7.45. In our experience, too much acid in the body diminishes the luster in skin and hair, interferes with muscle tone, makes the skin pallor gray and makes us look old before our time.

Many health experts, including Dr. Alejandro Junger (author of *Clean: The Revolutionary Program to Restore the Body's Natural Ability to Heal Itself),* believe that an acidic state is unhealthy for your bones. When your blood becomes too acidic from the foods you eat, your bones begin to release calcium into the bloodstream in an attempt to bring your body back to a healthier alkaline state, and this loss of calcium in the bones can lead to osteoporosis.

Here's how the acid/alkaline equation was described to us. Think of your insides as an aquarium. Initially, the water is clear and the fish frisky. As they're fed, the fish absorb some of their food and excrete the rest. The waste turns the water cloudy and acidic. If it's not cleaned, the fish become sick from swimming in the toxic environment. In the human digestive tract, fruits and vegetables help sweep waste from our systems. If we don't consume enough of them, waste can remain in our colon and bloodstream and elevate our acidity level. The more acidic we become, the more oxygen is driven from the body, and the more susceptible we are to disease. Among the diseases known to thrive in an acid environment are diabetes, high cholesterol, acid reflux, gout, heartburn, osteoporosis and even cancer. Sugars and processed carbohydrates and too much protein, coffee, alcohol and soft drinks increase acid levels.

Although it may seem counterintuitive, there are some foods you might think are acidic—and you'd be right—but when they're eaten, they ignite a digestive reaction that is alkalizing to the body. Foods with "weak acids"—like fresh lemon, raw apple cider vinegar and cultured or fermented dairy foods such as yogurt, kefir and fermented vegetables or kimchi—trigger the pancreas to produce the alkaline substance bicarbonate (as in baking soda), which neutralizes acid. The body absorbs the bicarbonate and becomes more alkaline. Green juices, exploding with nutrition, are excellent for alkalizing the body. (See more on Green Superfoods later in this chapter.)

Deep breathing also promotes alkalinity, and when we sleep, our bodies go through what's called an "alkaline tide"—as it becomes more alkaline, enzymes that eliminate waste from our organs and bloodstream are activated (another reason it's crucial to get the right amount of sleep). In the morning we tend to be acidic from cleansing and healing all night, and the acid needs to be released through elimination. That is why it is important to choose wisely what you eat or drink first thing in the morning. We recommend drinking water upon rising and then continuing with a green juice.

The Importance of Enzymes

Enzymes are protein molecules produced by living organisms that catalyze (set in motion) specific biochemical reactions. When you breathe, when you salivate, when you digest, you have enzymes to thank. These worker bees construct, synthesize and create a molecular charge that turns food into viable energy. Different enzymes are needed for different kinds of nutrients (fat, protein, sugars, etc.) in order to convert what you are eating into energy. As we age, our enzyme levels decline. This is due to the body being robbed of its own natural enzymes from eating what we call non-foods. You may notice as you get older that you're less able to tolerate the spicy foods you love or that you don't recover as quickly from the aches and pains of weekend sports. This reduced vitality and stamina can be a sign that your enzyme levels are low.

Fast food and too much fat and sugar require excessive amounts of enzymes to be digested. The cellular impact of stress and environmental pollution results in our enzyme-making machinery having to work overtime to mitigate the damage. Many researchers now view the aging process and death itself as the endgame of diminished enzyme potential; the human organism can no longer repair and maintain itself.

The good news is that we can slow down this trend by eating foods that are high in enzymes, including fresh papaya, pineapple, mango, kiwi, sprouts, raw seeds, and nuts soaked in water (and refrigerated after draining). Raw foods are high in enzymes. In fact, a major tenet for raw foodists is the fact that they don't heat the enzymes out of their foods, which makes the food more digestible. We also like to fortify ourselves with supplemental food-based enzymes, which can be found at health food stores or online.

Green Superfoods

Superfoods got their label because they're packed with nutrition rather than with calories. Green superfoods—kale, spinach and other leafy greens, as well as barley and wheat grasses, wild blue green algae, spirulina and chlorella—are an alkalinizing part of our daily diet. We make shakes with them in the morning and oftentimes throughout the day. They are very easy to digest and assimilate, so the nutrition immediately goes into the bloodstream and feeds the body.

Check out www.foodmatters.tv for a good description of green superfoods and what they can do. In short, they help oxygenate the blood, burn fat, aid digestion and stimulate the metabolism. Barley grass, for example, has 11 times more calcium than cow's milk, 5 times more iron than spinach and 7 times more vitamin C than orange juice. Not only is it a superfood, it's also a bit of a superhero!

> *Mariel: We plant a garden every year. We are careful to get great soil from a wonderful old guy who is a master composter. The more we learn about soil, the more intrigued we are with our garden and the connection the soil has to its productivity. We are so excited every day to see what has grown—how HUGE the zucchinis are and how diverse our tomato plants seem to be. Every day is a new discovery. We also love that we can plant in a fairly small amount of space and get a large bounty from it. I tweet about my garden and, of course, the chickens ("the girls") all the time.*

Free Radicals and Antioxidants

As mentioned earlier, free radicals are non-stabilized molecules. They have an extra, unpaired electron, and in their search for a complementary ion, they destabilize other healthy molecules. These cellular spoilers cause a chain reaction of destruction, which, if not arrested, can lead to illness and disease.

Free radicals are cellular renegades running riot, and antioxidants are the body's protectors; they are designed to restore homeostasis to cells where the free radicals have caused imbalance. The body gets antioxidants, which include vitamins A, C and E, beta-carotene (found in orange and yellow fruits and veggies) and selenium from food (and food-based supplements if you are not getting proper nutrition). Foods rich in antioxidants include blueberries, blackberries, Peruvian potatoes, watermelon, papaya, pink grapefruit, leafy greens, green tea, red wine and dark chocolate (the darker the better, but *even* better is cacao). When it comes to the wine (whose antioxidant is resveratrol) and chocolate, remember that a little goes a long way. (It's important to note that in the right quantity or balance, free radicals are healthy and can help fight illness. It's only when they proliferate that they become dangerous to the body.) As with everything, whether it's acid or alkaline, free radicals or antioxidants, the important thing is to strive for a healthy balance that keeps the body in harmony and working properly.

Mariel: When it comes to making new choices, especially in food, there are different approaches. If you are like me, you'll like changing one or two things at a time. I know I'm more successful this way. When people say they want to change the way they eat, I say, "Change your breakfast." Bobby, on the other hand, takes a much more aggressive approach to change, and that works for him. His attitude is, "You want change? Then change! Change everything. Just do it or I'll tie you to a tree and do it for you!" We have much more power and capability than we ever give ourselves credit for. If only we could see this, we would never limit ourselves as much as we do. Nevertheless, we know everyone is different and encourage you to find what is a comfortable stretch for you.

Magical Coconuts

As we said before, whenever possible we try to buy our food locally, but coconuts are one of the few exceptions we make. These fruits are nutritional powerhouses, but they don't grow around California where we live. The meat and oil in coconuts are antioxidant rich and also have antiviral properties. In fact, they are currently being studied for use in fighting HIV/AIDS and Alzheimer's disease.

Coconut oil is great for cooking because it can withstand high heat without breaking down and forming trans fats like some other vegetable oils. And coconut water is a fantastic hydrator. Because its electrolyte structure so closely matches that of human blood, it has been used in emergency IV drips. High in potassium and other minerals, but minus the unhealthy dyes and sugars in commercial sports drinks, coconut water is an ideal thirst quencher for workouts. There are many choices out there for coconut water. Don't be fooled by all of them. Most are heated and processed and say so in tiny lettering somewhere on the packaging. When coconut water is heated, it is not as good for you. It basically becomes sugar water. When raw, unheated and untreated, it retains all its healthy nutrients. We often buy coconut water frozen and let it thaw in our fridge.

> *Bobby: Coconut water is like algae. You can freeze it, then thaw it, and 80 to 90 percent of its properties will still be intact. There is also a high-pressure technique that a company called Harvest uses where thousands of pounds of pressure per square inch are applied to the coconuts in order to retain the chemical structure, nutrients and flavor when extracted. My complaint five years ago when coconut water started coming on the market here was, "What's it doing in a box? It stays on a shelf for a year? They pasteurized it!" Mariel and I use frozen coconut water. It's flash-frozen, really clean, and not pasteurized. Because of what we have learned in our own research, we've decided to avoid pasteurized foods as much as possible because the heating process destroys vital enzymes that enable them to be digested by the body.*

The Truth about Milk

Most of us have never enjoyed the luxury of a glass of raw milk the way it was meant to be—fresh from cows or goats that have been treated well and fed well. Instead we've grown up drinking milk that's been altered with additives and stripped of much of its natural nutrition, flavor and nutrients due to pasteurization and/or homogenization and often coming from factory farm-raised and abused cows and goats. Raw milk, according to some leading dairies that pasteurize, is superior to pasteurized milk. In a way, it comes down to clean milk vs. dirty milk in some cases. We've grown up with the idea that pasteurization (heating milk to eliminate bacteria and other nastiness) is essential for making milk safe for consumption. Not so.

Raw milk from responsible organic farms is pure, clean, nutrient-rich and safe to drink. In fact, certified raw milk must meet rigorous standards with regard to the feeding and health of the cows, methods of collecting the milk and composition of the milk itself. Buying raw milk can be tricky, depending on where you live, but in California and other states, sales are legal. Go to the Weston Price Foundation website for information about finding raw milk in your area. We drink raw milk and eat raw butter and raw milk cheeses.

If you leave a carton of pasteurized milk unrefrigerated, it will quickly go rancid. Non-refrigerated raw milk, on the other hand, can be turned into another food like kefir, which is a drinkable yogurt, or entirely edible sour cream. Despite the debates about drinking low-fat or non-fat milk, or even no milk at all, our research and experience have lead us to choose whole, full-fat, certified raw cow's milk. Raw milk contains all 22 of the essential amino acids, is loaded with its original unadulterated vitamins, minerals and proteins, is a complete food and contains beneficial bacteria that contribute to healthy digestion. The pasteurization process compromises every benefit that we can gain from consuming raw milk and milk products.

While we're talking about raw milk, we should reassure those of you who believe that whole dairy products will make you fat. A little-known fact: Raw dietary fat, whether dairy fat, coconut oil or avocadoes, doesn't turn into body fat. We drink raw milk and eat raw butter and raw milk cheeses—good food that is good for you—because they are rich, delicious and actually satisfy the appetite more easily so you don't eat as much.

As for those of you who think you're lactose intolerant, maybe you're not. We've convinced some friends and family members who thought they were lactose intolerant to try raw milk. They did and have had no adverse reactions. Some have even gone on to tolerate pasteurized milk and cheese after priming their systems with the enzymes and good bacteria in raw milk that is needed to help assimilate and digest the pasteurized along with the raw versions.

> *Bobby: Growing up I always had problems drinking milk. About 15 years ago, a friend of mine offered me a glass of raw milk, telling me how great it was for you. I told him I couldn't—I was lactose intolerant. He said, "Just try it." I did and, long story short, raw milk products are now a staple in my diet.*
>
> *Years later, the story repeated itself when I offered my friend Matt some raw milk. He said he was lactose intolerant and was even taking medication for it. If he ate a piece of pasteurized cheese, he'd double over in pain. I convinced him to have a glass of raw milk, just like my friend had convinced me years before. He drank a glass of milk with no adverse reaction, and twenty minutes later he drank another one and actually felt better from drinking it. Over a period of time, he was able to eat anything pasteurized that he wanted—cheese pizza, ice cream, no problem. The reason? Some whole food experts say it's because when you drink RAW milk, your gut becomes repopulated with the lactose enzymes and friendly bacteria that help the body digest the dairy. For me, raw milk is the way nature intended, especially when it comes from a clean farm where there are healthy cows with adequate housing and humane milking procedures. These requirements keep the nutrition impeccably high. That's simply the way I like it!*

Genetically Modified Organisms (GMOs)

GMO stands for "genetically modified organisms." These are plants or animals created through the gene-splicing techniques of biotechnology (also called genetic engineering, or GE). In the food world, GMOs are scientifically altered to produce specific attributes in crops—higher yields, thicker skin (making them easier to transport to market) and resistance to certain pests or drought. Sounds great, right? Proponents of GMOs say they even have the potential to address the issue of global hunger. Who doesn't want that? But here's the problem: GMOs designed for human consumption are believed by many to be linked to allergies, toxins, new diseases and nutritional problems. Most developed countries around the world, including Australia, Japan and all of the countries in the European Union, consider GMOs unsafe and have imposed significant restrictions or outright bans on the production and sale of GMOs. United States Food and Drug Administration (FDA) scientists have urged long-term safety studies of GMOs but have been ignored.

Besides their potential health hazards, GMOs create a scenario in which it is possible for world food production to become dominated by a few large companies, including Monsanto (currently the largest GMO seed producer). Farmers using GMO seeds cannot save and store their seeds for future sowing because the seeds are owned by the corporation and must be purchased again every year. What if GMO seeds blow into a neighboring field and contaminate a non-GMO crop? Farmers have been sued by Monsanto for this very reason. In fact, Monsanto filed 144 patent-infringement lawsuits against farmers between 1997 and April 2010. And those farmers whose crops are contaminated by GMO seeds are further impacted financially because many GMO crops cannot be sold to important export markets, such as Europe, China and Japan.

In technical terms, we think GMOs are creepy. What's even creepier is that there are no laws demanding that GMO ingredients be listed as such on food labels. An estimated 60 to 70 percent of the packaged goods lining supermarket shelves contain GMO products and no one knows it. We are big proponents of getting GMOs labeled on all foods from corn chips to dog food. More than 90 percent of the U.S. soybean crop is genetically modified, and nearly three-quarters of all corn planted in the U.S. is genetically modified. So if it comes in a can or a box and contains soybean oil or corn syrup, chances are it contains GMOs. This is another reason to shop at your local farmers market.

We are not science experiments. There has been no long-term human testing on GMOs. The U.S. and Canada are the only two large countries that have no labeling for genetically modified organisms. *No labels = no traceability of harmful effects = no liability.*

Testing in animals consuming GMOs has shown infertility, immune system suppression, accelerated aging, altered genetics and alterations in liver, kidney, spleen and gut function. And GMOs are creating "super weeds" that need more toxic pesticides, which destroys sustainable agriculture. Once this kind of farming takes place, the cycle of toxicity continues to expand.

If you'd like to learn more about the GMO controversy or get a list of foods that are less likely to contain GMOs, check out www.center forfoodsafety.org and www.truefoodnow.org.

Choose Your Food Carefully

If a food is classified as organic, it means that the food was raised or grown without the use of synthetic fertilizers or pesticides, sewage sludge, GMOs or ionizing radiation. Yep, large corporate farms do all that to our food . . . not cool. Farm animals that are used to produce organic products have not been fed antibiotics or growth hormones. Call us crazy—we think organic isn't just a better way but an *essential* way to eat if you want to be, feel and look your best.

Keep in mind when you're at the farmers market that applying for organic certification is an expensive undertaking. Some of that cost is passed on to the consumer. Also, many farmers adhere to organic practices without bothering to pay for the certification. So get to know your farmers. Even if they can't legally hang the *organic* banner outside their stall, their food may be spray- and pesticide-free . . . you just need to ask. Do your research wherever and whenever you buy your food. Sometimes local and sustainable is the best buy, and it's almost always the best choice for your health.

Mariel: My cookies, Blisscuits, are made with 40 percent organic ingredients. It is too expensive for my small company to use organic almonds because the almond market is subject to tremendous ups and downs. Even though they are not fully organic, the almonds in Blisscuits are not processed—no preservatives in them—so they're healthier than conventionally farmed almonds. The closer you get to the pure source, the more empowered you'll be. When reading labels, the rule of thumb is that simple is generally good for you. Buy organic when you can; it does make a difference. When you can't buy organic, at least buy unprocessed, spray-free and simple foods.

Protein Sources

When it comes to the vegetarian/vegan versus omnivore debate, only you can determine what is right for you. If you choose a vegetables-only route, just be sure that you're getting all the proteins and fats that your body needs. Knowledge and discipline are required to keep your body nourished and balanced on a vegetarian or vegan regimen and may not be ideal for everybody. Remember that your blood type, your lifestyle, your climate, your heritage and your environment need to be considered. If you are an A blood type, you may do great on a fully plant-based diet, similar to the vegetarians in India, but an O blood type may need more animal protein.

We're extremely active in our pursuit of physical, mental and emotional fitness, and after a lot of trial and error, we've worked out what is currently best for our bodies. We eat eggs, poultry and meat, but we're adamant about knowing how it was raised and killed. We believe that animal protein is part of the food chain, but eating humanely treated animals, raised and cared for ethically, is very different from eating terrorized animals from factory farms. Our rule is that we don't eat abused animals.

One of our favorite meats is bison. A traditional American Indian belief is that when you eat bison, you absorb its vitality and power. Bison is a lean meat, and lean protein helps your body create more lean muscle.

When it comes to fish, we *only* eat wild-caught, *never* farm-raised. Because farm-raised fish are raised in a controlled environment, they are unable to forage on a normal diet of crustaceans, plankton and algae, which give salmon its beautiful pinkish orange color. The flesh of farm-raised salmon, which are often fed GMO grain, antibiotics and carrots (we have certainly never heard of a carrot-eating salmon) is an unappealing gray. To make the salmon more marketable, salmon farmers choose a shade from a special color wheel (like at your local paint store) to help them add just the right amount of artificial dyes to their feed to achieve that perfect "natural" salmon color.

Wild salmon endure an amazing journey from where they spawn up river to sometimes thousands of miles (up to 2,000 miles recorded) to the ocean and back again, returning to nearly the exact place where they were born. Their swim gives them their color, their flavor and their intense vitality. We feel strongly about eating as close to the way Nature intended as possible. Eating wild fish rather than farm-raised is one way we honor our convictions and honor the delicate balance of Nature's right of passage.

Mariel: I was vegan for 16 years, and though I do well eating mostly vegetables, I came to realize I need animal protein. When I think about how I grew up, I ate grass-fed beef and game that my father hunted. We ate farm-fresh eggs and local cheese. I realized after my bout with veganism that I was more vital as a kid because I ate in a way that suited my body type and activity level and ultimately my ethics. Bobby and I are adamant that every person is different and that what serves one doesn't necessarily serve another. We love our food and love that a lot of it we produce ourselves. We eat eggs from our own chickens and drink organic raw goat or cow milk from a neighbor's farm.

Bobby: Growing up, I ate anything and just about everything. I am the guy who can eat a pair of shoes and digest them! My grandparents had farms and gardens. When the farms were gone and the gardens diminished, I discovered fast food. It was convenient. I realized in my mid 30s that making fast food a way of life was just a fast way to shorten my life. Hell, I couldn't even breathe out of my nose, and my body was plugged up. Every organ was sluggish, and all my tissues were toxic. Making adjustments to my food, water and lifestyle gave me the opportunity to thrive! Today I eat a combination of live, cooked, raw or sprouted foods that are clean and powerful. Growing younger and living disease-free is an amazing accomplishment.

The Scoop on Sugar

The average American consumes more than 100 pounds of sugar a year. That's insane. Sugar is at the very tip of our personal food pyramid, meaning it's the food we recommend eating least. Sweet foods can be a source of great joy if you can eat them in moderation, but white sugar is addictive. This is just one reason food companies load it into their products, making even savory foods addictive. (Artificial sweeteners are not the answer either, by the way. Check out *New York Times* bestselling author Dr. Joseph Mercola's book *Sweet Deception* for more on the studies regarding the popular artificial sweeteners Splenda, NutraSweet and Equal.)

The more we eat sugar, the more we want it. Many people actually eat sugar in their breakfast, lunch, dinner and snacks . . . every single day of the week. They eat it virtually all day long. It's a serious problem. If they go without sugar for any length of time, they begin to crave it. If you can relate, it's time to break free from your sugar addiction.

Think of sugar as something to enjoy when you celebrate special occasions. When we were kids, of course we ate dessert, but it wasn't every night or every day. Apple pies, cakes and cookies happened at Sunday dinners, birthdays or with guests. They were often homemade and filled with love. And we looked forward to them all week long. And on most nights if you needed something sweet, dessert was a piece of fruit. When you eat a peach in season, the sweetness is perfect and that craving is satiated. You appreciate treats far more when you make them special!

For those of you who have a love/hate relationship with sugar and you punish yourself when you splurge on a sweet (which often leads to eating ten times a single serving), instead of berating yourself, give yourself permission to relish it. That way you are more likely not to overindulge. On regular days, when cake, pie and cookies are not the best choice, eat fresh seasonal fruit, desserts made with raw honey or simply berries in season. If you want chocolate, for example, make it the simplest, purest form you can find—not a commercial candy bar with all its additives and chemicals, but a decadent dark chocolate whose emphasis is the super nutrient-dense cacao and not sugar. Savor it!

A note about RAW HONEY . . . this is a healing food like no other. When unheated and untreated, raw honey is 90 percent enzymes, meaning it helps your body with digestion, and only 10 percent sugar or carbohydrate. If you heat honey in baked goods, for example, or put it into hot beverages, that ratio is inverted and becomes only 10 percent enzymes and 90 percent sugar (having a detrimental effect on your glycemic index). Make RAW honey part of your diet—it aids in digestion, helps fight allergies and lessens your sugar cravings as well.

Mariel: When it comes to sugar, I don't seem to have an off switch. Although I eat a lot of fruit, I haven't eaten white sugar or its products in years. I know myself and know that I would rather not eat a food that is addictive in nature because I have had, in the past, a tendency to overeat them. I stay away from processed sugar, but it doesn't mean I stay away from sweet treats. Bobby and I create raw desserts or baked goods made with Xylitol or Stevia instead of sugar. We whip raw cream and add raw honey and vanilla extract to it, then we spoon it over seasonal berries—unbelievably yummy! The truth is, I prefer to binge on salad. The amount of salad I eat blows Bobby away. I can eat more greens than a cow. It's nutty! But he can eat the same amount of raw meat. We think that balances us!

Mindful Eating

Another really important thing to keep in mind about food is to make it your friend by creating a mindful practice around it. When you're eating, concentrate on eating. Turn off the TV, ditch the crackBerry or iPad, sit at the table, and pay attention to each mouthful. If you're used to eating while you're doing something else, this will be a whole new experience for you. You'll be in touch with your body and all of your senses. You'll feel the texture of the food in your mouth. You'll become aware of how much you chew before swallowing. And you'll feel your sense of fullness coming on before you've gone too far. This is a great technique if you're trying to lose weight and want to stop overeating. Eating mindfully also becomes a part of deepening your awareness of who you are; it's one more way to be present in the moment.

> *Bobby: This morning I was busy, so for breakfast I blended four raw eggs, a pint of blueberries, bee pollen, raw honey, raw goat milk, raw whey, raw coconut water and walnuts and made a smoothie. I also had two pieces of natural probiotic sourdough toast with raw butter. A smoothie packed with nutrient-rich ingredients paired with a healthy bread choice makes a great breakfast on the go.*

Salt and Processed Foods

It's been estimated that 60 percent of the average American's diet consists of processed foods: potato chips, cookies, cakes, lunch meats, bacon, canned soups, stews and sauces—anything that's been fiddled with in a factory, pumped up with unpronounceable ingredients and packaged to last a few lifetimes on a supermarket shelf. In other words, for the average American, the healthy food pyramid has been turned upside down. No wonder our healthcare costs are astronomical.

Processed foods are loaded with refined salts. In 2010, *Time* magazine estimated that the average American eats 3,500 mgs of salt a day, about 80 percent of it from processed food. The American Heart Association recommends a maximum of 1,500 to 2,300 mgs a day. The dangers of excess sodium chloride from the kind of salt found in processed foods—and on the tables of most kitchens—are legion: high blood pressure, strokes, poor kidney function, depression and loss of calcium, which puts bone health at risk.

We don't believe all salt is bad. Sodium chloride is essential for animal life, but it is harmful in excess. And it is the oldest, most universal food seasoning. All living creatures need the sodium and chloride in small amounts. It helps carry nutrients to our cells, and it regulates water and fluid balance in the body. The sodium ion itself is used for electrical signaling in the nervous system, facilitating the transmission of nerve impulses. It's found naturally in fruits and vegetables, and we couldn't live without it. Then why has salt, as most of us know it, been getting such a bad rap?

There are two camps on this issue: one, which includes the medical establishment, doesn't recognize the difference between refined salt and unrefined salt. Both, they say, are sodium chloride. End of story. The other camp, the one where we pitch our tent along with Dr. Mercola and other nutrition experts, says that refined salt and unrefined salt are worlds apart. Refined salt is heated to make it recrystallize and chemically treated to keep it bright white, non-clumping and easy to pour. All trace minerals are washed away in the process, and the resulting product is 97.5 percent sodium chloride and 2.5 percent added chemicals, including iodine and moisture absorbers.

Unrefined sea salt by contrast is 84 percent chloride and 16 percent minerals. It's usually grayish and flaky (although Himalayan salt, dug from ancient seabeds, is pink). Unrefined sea salt is subject to clumping—big deal. Because it's natural, the body is programmed to work with it.

Real Salt, Celtic sea salt, Himalayan salt, and SEA90 (which we use in our swimming pool instead of chlorine, feed to our plants and sprinkle into our chicken feed) are prime examples of unrefined salts. (Not all sea salt is unrefined.) When Homer described salt as "a divine substance," this is what he was talking about. The Romans considered salt so valuable that our English word "salary" comes from the Latin *salarium*—the money Roman soldiers were given to purchase precious salt.

Good salt is extremely important for mineral intake, meaning that your body will absorb minerals better when you have it in your diet. It's vital for the proper functioning of the adrenal glands, which regulate many hormones. It helps replenish electrolytes and balance your system after exercise. If you go out for a long hike or do a lot of exercise, you can add a pinch of good salt to some pure water for a hydrating drink.

Table salt and the salt in processed and canned foods, on the other hand, wreak havoc on the body in high quantities and have been linked to high blood pressure, stroke and heart disease. Monosodium glutamate (MSG) is a form of salt often added to Chinese food and processed foods where it serves as a flavor enhancer and preservative. While the FDA says that MSG is generally safe, others maintain that it exerts a negative effect on blood sugar levels, which can lead to overeating. Many people have reported a variety of MSG-related reactions (referred to as MSG complex) ranging from headaches to nausea to chest pain. When checking labels, be on the lookout for "natural flavoring," sodium caseinate, maltodextrin and anything "hydrolyzed," as these become MSG in the system.

> *Mariel: I recently had major back pain and was unable to get to the bottom of it. In my running around looking for answers, I met with a chiropractor thinking I would get another severe cracking of my joints. But instead she did some muscle testing and found I was super dehydrated. I thought, "Oh, come on, I drink several quarts of water a day. There's no way I am dehydrated." But it turns out that the water I was drinking was not being properly absorbed into my system. She recommended that I drink a glass of water in the morning and one before bed with a teaspoon of Real Salt in them (Real Salt has the highest mineral count of all of the salts Bobby and I have looked into). All I can say is that it works. It took a couple of days and the pain went away. Now I drink my salty water every day!*

Herbs and Spices with Benefits

Now that we've given certain types of salt a clean bill of health, below is a list of other herbs and spices that have particular benefits. We recommend using organic spices, as this means that they have not been irradiated (exposed to radiation).

- Cayenne supports blood flow and metabolism. It is anti-inflammatory, helps produce saliva to aid in digestion and good oral health and is also a circulatory stimulant.

- Cinnamon boosts metabolism, regulates blood sugar, is good for the nervous system and is great for heart health.

- Dates, which are natural sweeteners, are good for thyroid health thanks to their rich selenium content.

- Flaxseed oil and flaxseeds, which can be sprinkled on salads, are good for the prostate; they are also excellent sources of mono-unsaturated fatty acids, including omega-3 and omega-6.

- Chlorella, kamut, and green superfood drinks alkalinize and oxygenate the body. These super greens help with chronically over-acidic pH in the body.

- Turmeric works as one of the most powerful anti-inflammatories (add a dash to a raw fat like whole yogurt for most effectiveness).

- Ginger is great for digestion and acts as an anti-inflammatory as well. It is also good for brain and lung function.

Consider planting your own herb garden or raising a few of your favorite herbs in pots on the patio or windowsill. Herbs like basil, mint, thyme and rosemary are easy to grow if you have enough sunlight. When you snip off leaves to cook with or toss into salads, you have the peace of mind of knowing where your spices came from and that they haven't been processed or sprayed with chemicals. Fresh herbs can make any meal delicious, but you can also buy your favorite herbs in bunches and dry them to use in your favorite dish when you don't have time to run to the market.

Develop Your Personal Good Food Habits

Now that we've given you an overall look at our view on food and covered some important nutrition information, it's time for you to start making it personal. How can you apply what we have shared with you to your everyday life in order to stay healthy and fit? We'll continue to talk about some of the foods we eat and how we prepare them, and we know that you will find your own unique inspiration as you browse through your local farmers market. Just remember, as *New York Times* bestselling author and food authority Michael Pollan puts it: "Eat food. Not too much. Mostly plants."

Breakfast sets the tone for the rest of the day. While you were sleeping, your body worked diligently to repair and rejuvenate itself. The best reward for all its hard work is something alkalinizing—clean water, green juice or an antioxidant-rich green tea are great ways to start the day and give your body what it needs. We often hike or work out before breakfast. When we do, we'll eat a more substantial breakfast, maybe an egg white omelet (see the recipe on page 93) or a bowl of steel-cut oats with fresh blueberries. For lunch, we'll usually have a big green salad—arugula, kale and various types of lettuce—often along with whatever protein was left over from dinner the night before, maybe some chicken, salmon or bison.

Then for dinner, we keep it simple. And we keep it early. We usually eat between 6:00 p.m. and 7:00 p.m., or a good rule of thumb is to eat before the sun sets if possible. We'll roast chicken or grill fish— or if we have bison on hand, we prepare it tartare-style or sear it on either side, leaving the center rare. We always have loads of vegetables and a big salad too.

It is easy to eat well when you understand how powerful food is to your well-being. Be excited to create food habits that suit your individuality and are simple and healing. Running with Nature is meant to be personalized, so you get to decide how you want to incorporate some of these food shifts into your life. Maybe you will decide to dive in headfirst, tossing all sugar, pasteurized dairy and maybe even the microwave into the trash this minute. Or maybe you will be more comfortable starting slowly with the elimination of one type of food and/or the inclusion of another. For example, maybe instead of reaching for a piece of white toast with jam at breakfast, you can substitute steel-cut oats with raw honey or blueberries. Always feel empowered knowing that your body is a map to your optimum health and *Running with Nature* is here as a support for your expedition.

Grand Canyon Railroad
(circa 1901) Williams,
Arizona. Christmas 2011.
(Photo by David Paul)

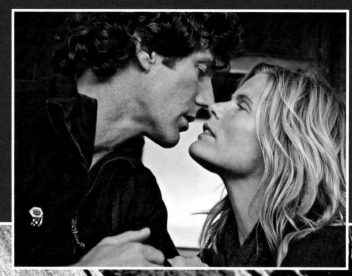

Climbing Needle and Spoon
Pywiack Dome 510 a-R 3rd
pitch. Tuolumne Meadows,
Yosemite, California, 2011.
(Photo by David Paul)

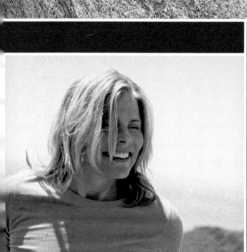

Mariel road tripping. Big Sur, California. 2012.
Photo by Boone Speed)

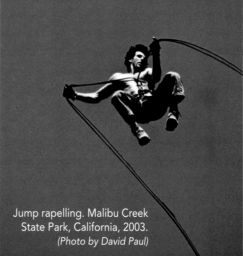

Jump rapelling. Malibu Creek
State Park, California, 2003.
(Photo by David Paul)

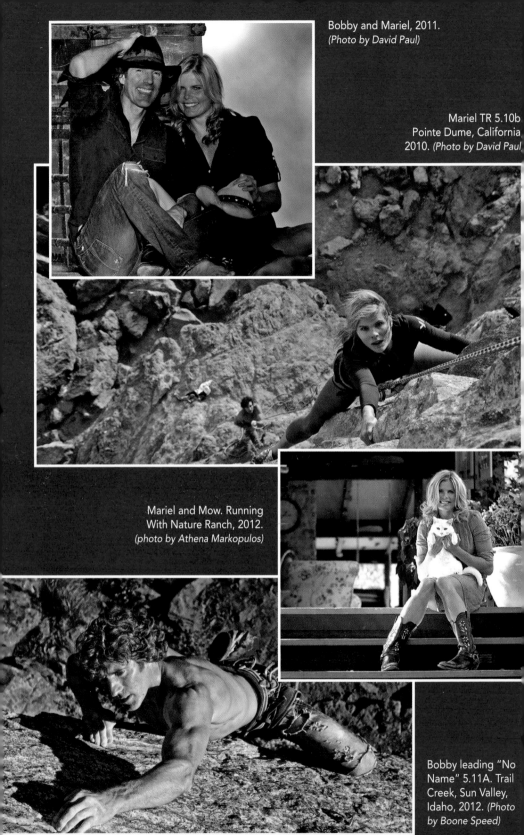

Bobby and Mariel, 2011.
(Photo by David Paul)

Mariel TR 5.10b
Pointe Dume, California
2010. *(Photo by David Paul)*

Mariel and Mow. Running
With Nature Ranch, 2012.
(photo by Athena Markopulos)

Bobby leading "No
Name" 5.11A. Trail
Creek, Sun Valley,
Idaho, 2012. *(Photo
by Boone Speed)*

Bobby and Mariel. Sunrise at Grand Canyon, Arizona, Christmas 2011. *(Photo by David Paul)*

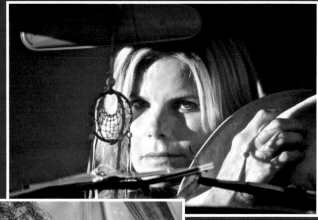

Mariel.
'57 Studebaker, 2011.
(Photo by David Paul)

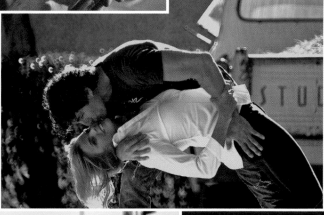

Bobby.
'57 Studebaker, 2011.
(Photo by David Paul)

The Kiss.
'57 Studebaker, 2011.
(Photo by David Paul)

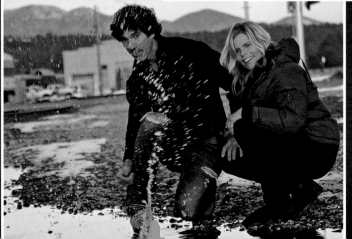

Bobby and Mariel. Grand
Canyon Railroad, Christmas
2010. (Photo by David Paul)

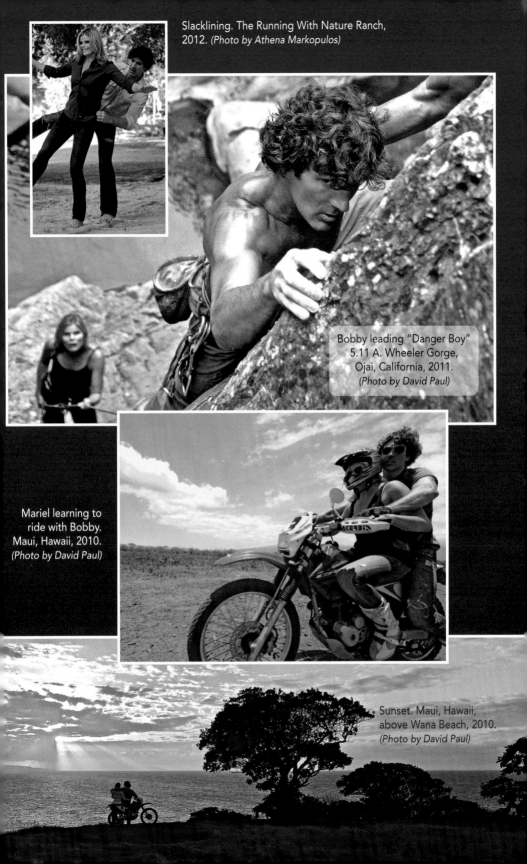

Slacklining. The Running With Nature Ranch, 2012. *(Photo by Athena Markopulos)*

Bobby leading "Danger Boy" 5.11 A. Wheeler Gorge, Ojai, California, 2011. *(Photo by David Paul)*

Mariel learning to ride with Bobby. Maui, Hawaii, 2010. *(Photo by David Paul)*

Sunset. Maui, Hawaii, above Wana Beach, 2010. *(Photo by David Paul)*

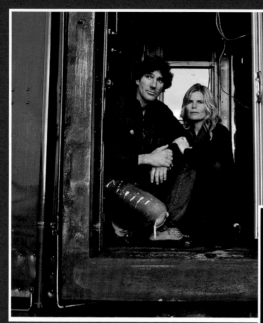

Mariel and Bobby,
Grand Canyon Railroad.
Williams, Arizona,
Christmas 2011.
(Photo by David Paul)

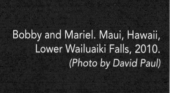

Bobby and Mariel. Maui, Hawaii,
Lower Wailuaiki Falls, 2010.
(Photo by David Paul)

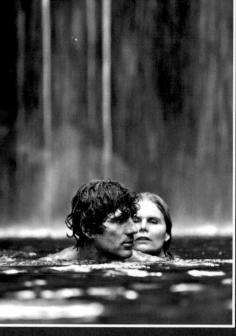

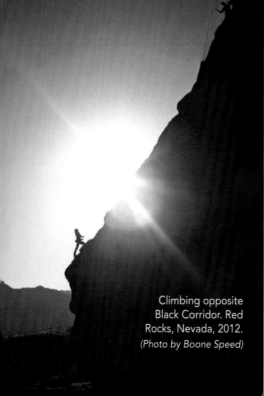

Climbing opposite
Black Corridor. Red
Rocks, Nevada, 2012.
(Photo by Boone Speed)

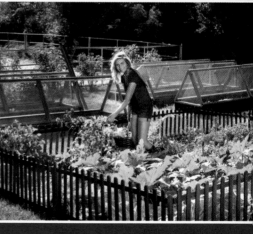

Mariel in the garden.
Running With Nature Ranch, 2011

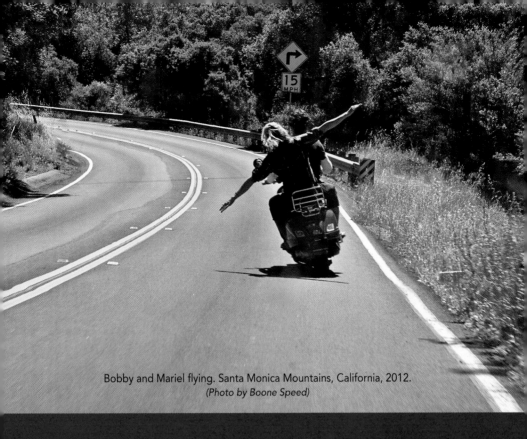

Bobby and Mariel flying. Santa Monica Mountains, California, 2012.
(Photo by Boone Speed)

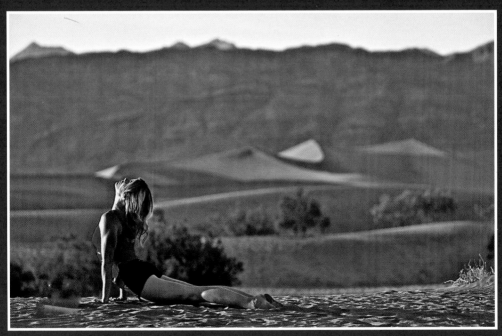

Mariel doing yoga at sunset. Sand dunes of Death Valley, 2012.
(Photo by Boone Speed)

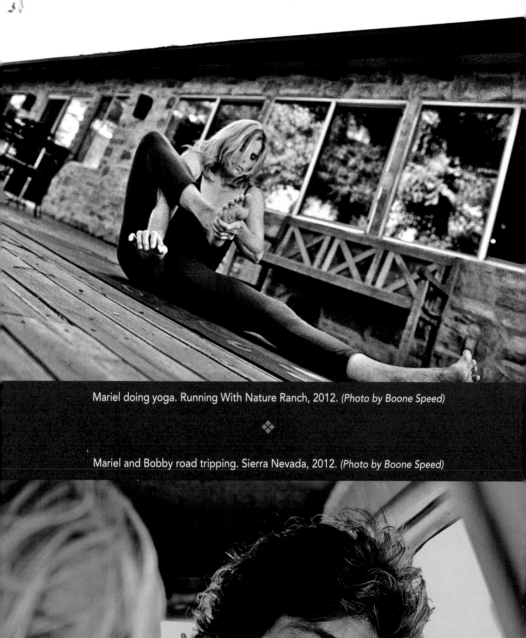

Mariel doing yoga. Running With Nature Ranch, 2012. *(Photo by Boone Speed)*

❖

Mariel and Bobby road tripping. Sierra Nevada, 2012. *(Photo by Boone Speed)*

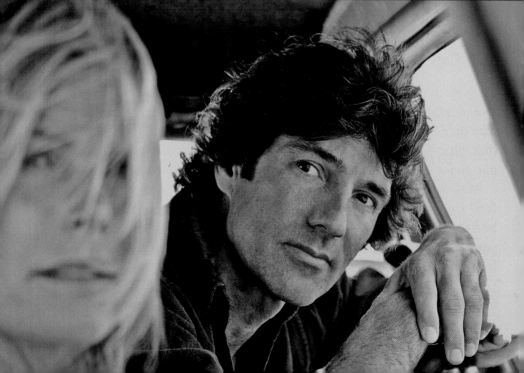

The best way to succeed at changing a habit is through planning and preparation. You transition to a more nutritious, healthy and happy you by having good food choices within easy reach when you're hungry.

Here are some helpful tips:

◆ Chop up vegetables—carrots, celery, green beans, peppers, radishes, jicama—and keep them in the fridge where you can grab them when you need a quick pick-me-up.

◆ Purge your pantry of the chips, the cookies, and all the other processed foods you know aren't good for you. It's easier to ignore something that's not there than to resist something that's staring you down from the cabinet!

◆ Keep plenty of fruit on hand. When your sweet tooth acts up, reach for berries, an apple, some seasonal citrus or bananas. And remember to choose bananas that are slightly green on the ends; when they are overripe, they are too high in sugar and have lost their high nutrient count.

◆ If you don't have a blender (we couldn't live without our Vitamix) get one. You can make filling and nutritious smoothies with endless fresh ingredients.

You Can Choose to Change

The mind is, by nature, resistant to change. As you establish your intention to improve your eating habits, it may play tricks on you. It may tempt you into believing that eating healthily is a deprivation and that what you really need to be happy and alert at 4:00 p.m. is a Twix bar and a Coke. Repeat after us: "That is a lie."

Make a decision right now that you will make better choices in food from this moment forward because you can and because you will be better on every level because of it. This is your body, your health, your life, and if you want to be the best YOU you can be, it will come from making the right choices. See food as your ally, your doctor and your friend . . . it is not a substitute for love, but it is healing when it is made from love. Take charge of your food and you will take charge of your life.

There's an old Zen proverb: "Before enlightenment, chop wood, carry water. After enlightenment, chop wood, carry water." Turn the preparation of your food into a mindful practice. By becoming fully present in any task, by feeling the action of it, becoming one with it, you lighten the "work" aspect and expand your state of awareness. Even simple things become rewarding. Make them ceremonial, make them important, and focus solely on them. As you do, you will discover what it means to connect to YOU.

We know this chapter on healthy eating contains a lot of information to wrap your head around. All good things become second nature in time. Start now and try a couple of our breakfast recipes. ENJOY!

Green Drink for Two

INGREDIENTS

kale leaves

$1/2$ avocado

1 raw date

2 tablespoons raw olive oil

2 teaspoons fresh turmeric or 1 teaspoon powdered

*1 heaping tablespoon raw honey
(unheated and untreated)*

*2 tablespoons Organic Lives Supergreens Powder
(available at opensky.com/marielhemingway)*

Dash of cinnamon

DIRECTIONS: Throw all ingredients into your Vitamix or other blender, whiz until well combined, then pour into tall drinking glasses and enjoy!

Egg White Omelet
with Avocado Yolk Sauce

INGREDIENTS

For the Omelet

Raw coconut oil for pan

$1/3$ cup organic local egg whites
(or Eggology organic egg whites)

Handful spinach leaves

Dash Real Salt

Black pepper to taste

For the Sauce

2–3 egg yolks

$1/2$ avocado

$1/2$ teaspoon turmeric

Dash Real Salt

Black and cayenne pepper, to taste

DIRECTIONS: To make the sauce, blend the yolks, avocado, turmeric, salt and peppers (a little cayenne goes a long way!) in a bowl with a fork.

To make the omelet, heat a medium-sized frying pan over *low* heat. Add enough coconut oil to coat bottom of pan. Pour in egg whites. When they turn from translucent to white, add Real Salt, pepper and spinach. Cover pan with lid until spinach has wilted and the whites are light and fluffy. Remove from heat.

Divide the egg white omelet between two plates. Pour half the sauce over each serving. To serve: You can add a simple romaine salad on the side, or if more starch is in order, try gluten-free sprouted bread or corn tortillas.

POINT-EARNING ACTIVITIES CHECKLIST

EAT WHOLESOME FOOD

- Take a look through your fridge and cabinets and toss at least two non-nutritious items. Easy targets include white sugar, white flour and processed junk food. Two things thrown away equals five points; four things thrown away equals ten points, and so on. Make the decision that when you throw them away, you agree not to eat those foods again.   **10 POINTS**

- Go to your local farmers market and stock up on fresh produce. Choose one new organic fruit or vegetable to try this week.   **10 POINTS**

  (Give yourself five extra points each week for trying a new fruit and vegetable. Remember, it has to be *new*.)

- Buy one or more whole herb plants and create a windowsill garden.   **10 POINTS**

- Chop up carrots, celery, peppers and other vegetables and have them in the fridge ready for snacking.   **10 POINTS**

- Check out the Weston Price Foundation and see if you can find raw (unpasteurized) milk, cheese, butter and yogurt in your area.   **10 POINTS**

- Include one or two enzyme-rich foods in your daily meals—raw vegetables and fruits and raw, unheated, untreated honey are a good start. Or try a fermented food (yogurt, kimchi, sauerkraut) with a meal.   **10 POINTS**

- Try a week without black tea or coffee and see how you feel. Try green tea or yerba mate as a substitute.   **10 POINTS**

- When you feel a sugar craving coming on, reach for something good for you—an apple, sprouted-bread toast with raw honey or raw nut butter, or berries.   **10 POINTS**

- Toss the iodized salt and replace it with natural unrefined sea salt or *Real Salt*. (This is our preference, but Celtic sea salt and Himalayan salt are good as well; check out options in your market.)   **10 POINTS**

- While you're eating, be mindful. Think about the food you're taking into your body. Slow down and be grateful. Chew your food slowly.   **10 POINTS**

TOTAL POINTS _____

CHAPTER 6

DRINK PURE WATER

"Life in us is like the water in a river."
—HENRY DAVID THOREAU

Water is symbolic of our state of well-being. In water there is clarity, fluidity and ease. Even when a river flows over rocks or dams and into oceans, it is always comprised of graceful movement. If we can see the state of our being as mirroring the natural mellifluous current of a river, we are able to relate to everything with more flexibility. Water has no hard corners or rigid edges, though it crashes into the jagged edges of rocks and other obstacles in its path while retaining its complete identity. Water represents the life force that flows through every one of us. Begin to see water as a metaphor for your life—a running river negotiating the eddies, the turns, the ripples and the rapids with grace. Without water we dry up. With an abundance of water, we flourish.

Water Is Life

Adults are made up of about 60 to 70 percent water, teens about 75 percent, and children 75 to 80 percent, while infants are made up of sometimes as much as 90 percent water. That is some serious fluid content. So it makes sense to begin looking at water as part of who you are. Water has the power to heal, protect and enhance your body and mind.

Water is essential to all forms of life on the planet, from trees to humans. Two-thirds of the earth is covered in water. Water sustains life. While we can go for weeks with no food, humans cannot live more than several days without water. We use it for everything—from drinking, bathing, playing, cooking and cleaning to staving off illness, eliminating toxins and coordinating motor and nerve function. Without water, our mucous membranes, which trap disease-causing microbes before they can do their dirty work, can't function. We would be unable to swallow, digest or eliminate. It's almost silly to say what we couldn't do without water, because the fact is, we couldn't do anything.

Water is essential for every chemical reaction throughout the body. Water enables our blood to carry nutrients and oxygen, helps to maintain our proper pH level and allows our kidneys to perform their crucial cleansing function. Our lymph system is similar to a small river winding through our bodies, cleansing every cell. Proper hydration allows that river to flow as it should.

We believe that water is one of the most underrated, overlooked medicines. Native Americans call water the medicine that heals all. So many minor ailments are caused by not drinking enough water—headaches, body aches, low energy, excess appetite, digestive problems, constipation, asthma and allergies, depression. When water corrects dehydration of the cells, healing is possible. Along with air, it is the simplest healer we can put in our bodies.

Start Your Day With Water . . .

And continue drinking all day long. It's the closest thing to a true fountain of youth, health and beauty.

After a night of fasting and accumulating toxins, drinking water first thing in the morning flushes out the buildup of impurities. It purifies your colon, making it a lot easier to absorb the nutrients in the *"good food"* you will be eating for the rest of the day. It increases the production of new blood and muscle cells. Water helps balance the lymph system, enabling it to regulate your fluid levels while fighting infection.

Ever wondered why people in humid climates have great skin? You guessed it . . . water. They are absorbing moisture from their environment. When taken internally, water does the same thing—it heightens the glow that comes from youthful-looking skin. Remember to drink a nice tall glass of water first thing in the morning to replenish the hydration your skin has lost during the night.

And finally, starting your day with water helps with weight loss. Drinking eight ounces of chilled water in the morning can boost your metabolism by 24 percent. And there's another way water helps with weight loss. Often when our body tells us to drink water by making us thirsty, we misunderstand the signal. Then, rather than pour ourselves a glass of water, we reach for something to eat. The next time you get what you think is a hunger pang, try drinking a big glass of water to see if your hunger disappears.

How Much Water Is Enough?

Virtually everyone has heard that the daily recommended intake of water is eight 8-ounce glasses a day. While this is probably a good rule of thumb, we generally believe that the right amount is different for everyone. For example, Mariel, at 135 pounds, needs approximately 85 ounces of water a day, and Bobby, at 200 pounds, needs approximately 120 ounces of water. Weight, environment, humidity, temperature, elevation and activity level all play a role in the amount of water we need to consume. You can also figure out your recommended daily water intake at www.nutrition.about.com/library/blwatercalculator .htm.

If you're working out all the time and losing water through perspiration, you'll need more water to keep properly hydrated. When we're out climbing, hiking or biking, we definitely need to drink more water than when we're just taking it easy. Of course, that sounds elementary, but it's surprising how easily we can forget to continue hydrating even after we cool down from a workout.

Dehydration and Athletic Performance

Water allows our bodies to function and recover properly when we engage in any intense or long-term physical activity such as sports or exercise. These activities create heat and loss of fluids. At the same time, believe it or not, they also suppress your thirst response. So make it a habit to drink plenty of fluids before, during and after any prolonged or intense physical activity.

The loss of fluids impairs physical and mental performance. A loss of fluid equaling 2 percent of a person's body weight can reduce performance by 10 to 20 percent. Without replenishing these fluids, a chain reaction is set off in a person's body that includes symptoms of early fatigue and impaired reaction time, judgment, concentration and decision-making. If an athlete loses just 1.5 quarts of water, he or she will suffer a 25 percent loss in stamina. This means they will ultimately have to put in more effort and get less results while being more prone to injury.

Because we tend to underestimate how much water we lose during physical activity, especially those of us who compete or engage in intense workouts regularly, it is important to make rehydration a priority. It's as simple as this—to make sure you're performing to your maximum potential, drink plenty of liquids before, during and after physical activity, even if you don't feel thirsty.

Warm Water Versus Cold Water

If you've been exercising and are overheated and thirsty, it's best to drink water that's a few degrees cooler than the temperature of your environment. Although it seems counterintuitive, cold water is passed through your stomach more quickly than warm, so it gets to your intestines and is absorbed more quickly. Along with hydrating the body, it will help bring your temperature down to a healthy level. We don't recommend shocking your system with ice water but rather with a slightly cool drink. Your body temperature is 98.6°F, remember, and there's no need to punish it with an arctic onslaught! In Chinese medicine, ice-cold beverages are believed to be hard on the spleen and kidneys, making them weak. This is why we ask for water with no ice when we go out to restaurants.

Especially in colder weather, it makes sense to drink warm drinks, including warm water, and to enjoy hot soups, stews and cooked foods. This is a natural way to create an internal heater for your body. It makes seasonal sense!

Beware of the Bottle

Even though most Americans don't manage to drink the advised eight glasses a day, we're tossing back a lot of water—more than 8 billion gallons a year. The question is whether we're drinking the *right* water. Every year, Americans put away an average 28.5 gallons of bottled water each, which translates to billions of discarded plastic bottles— 75 percent of which aren't recycled. According to Peter Gleick, author of *Bottled and Sold,* every second of every day 1,000 plastic water bottles are tossed out. According to the Pacific Institute, it takes about three liters of water to produce one liter of bottled water. Not to mention, plastic water bottle manufacturers generate more than 2.5 million tons of carbon dioxide a year and use over 17 million barrels of oil in the production process. So an act as simple as drinking water can, cumulatively, have a disastrous impact on the planet. Those pristine-looking bottles, by the way, are owned by big industry. Coke owns Dasani, PepsiCo owns Aquafina, and Nestle owns Pure Life. Just saying.

And the big catch is that store-bought water isn't necessarily any healthier than tap (which we'll get to in a moment). Bottled water has no chlorine, meaning that if bacteria are present when it's packaged, they can proliferate.

"There's no guarantee that bottled water is any safer than the water that comes out of your tap," says Wendy Gordon of the Natural Resources Defense Council. Tap water—which makes up 25 percent of bottled water, according to the Council—is subject to stricter standards and more rigorous testing than bottled water. In fact, bottled water that isn't shipped across state lines (about 79 percent of what's on the market) isn't subject to any standards at all. Researchers have found traces of fecal and glass matter, yeast and coliforms (bacteria) in some bottled water. Yuck!

Even if the water goes into a plastic bottle in pristine condition, that's not the end of the story. The plastic itself, especially when exposed to heat, is a problem (how many times have you left your water in the car on a summer day?), potentially shedding nasty chemicals into your drink.

You can't swallow the water companies' marketing jargon whole. Just because the bottle is labeled "natural" doesn't mean it's from a spring. A four-year study by the National Resources Defense Council found that 25 percent or more of bottled water is actually just bottled tap water, sometimes treated and sometimes not. Fluoride, which researchers now believe can be harmful (particularly to children and fetuses) at chronic low levels, can be added to water without being listed on the label.

Knowing where your water comes from is like knowing where your food is grown. We particularly like O2Cool Oxygen Water (full disclosure, Mariel is a spokesperson for them). This refreshing water is slightly alkaline and really does come from a natural sweet water spring (*sweet water* means that it is a naturally magnesium-rich spring) from Northern California. We also drink Noah's Water, which comes from the same source.

As always, if you do buy your water in bottles, buy local water. The NRDC estimates that some 4,000 tons of carbon dioxide are created by flying water in to the United States from Italy, France and Fiji. That's a huge carbon footprint.

The Tap Dance

Tap-water safety has been a topic of heated debate for decades. It's been found to contain thousands of chemicals, only 91 of which are tested for under the Safe Water Drinking Act, a federal law that hasn't been updated since 2000. Tap water hosts everything from chlorine to hormones to pharmaceuticals, some of which are flushed down toilets and contaminate the water supply. One research study by the Environmental Working Group (EWG) found traces of pesticides, heavy metals and industrial pollutants in tap water tested throughout the United States. The EWG study discovered many of the same pollutants in bottled water that they found in tap. Freaky, right?

Many municipal water systems treat their water with fluoride, a practice that began in the 1940s in an effort to combat tooth decay. With the advances in toothpaste, we no longer need fluoride in our water—its dental benefits come not from drinking it, but from its application to the teeth themselves. And, as we said earlier, scientists have found that prolonged ingestion of low doses of fluoride can have a negative health effect on everyone, especially children.

The good news is that a home filter can purify your tap water before it gets to you. If you can afford it, we highly recommend investing in a home filtration system that will filter the water coming out of every faucet in your home. The very best are carbon filters, and there are many that are highly recommended on the Greener Choices Consumer Reports website. Carbon filters snatch the contaminants out of water as it passes through. The slower the water, the more efficient the filters can be, so keep that in mind when you regulate the flow. (Steer clear of filters that contain methylene blue; studies are being done on its toxic potential, so why take the chance?)

You can also attach filters directly to your faucets. This is a less expensive way to go and may be more feasible for you. Keep in mind that the skin is the largest organ in our bodies and also the largest absorption vehicle. So bathing in water containing chlorine and whatever else is in your city water is not a good idea. That is why we travel with faucet filters (and recommend them for your showers if you can't afford a whole house water-filtration system). We want to be sure that the water we bathe in is merely cleaning us, not harming us.

Distilled, Vitalized and Alkaline Water

Distilled water is empty water—void of chemicals and minerals. So while it's not harmful, as your go-to drinking water it's less beneficial than water with minerals. (The lack of minerals makes it good for the teapot because it won't leave a mineral buildup.) This neutral state also makes it great for detoxing or for use when taking herbal medicine because it doesn't contain any properties that would conflict with the herb's chemistry. Also, distilled water is good for use in a neti pot (an Indian nasal teapot that flushes the sinuses with water and salt).

We put our filtered water and sometimes distilled water into the Vitalizer Plus, which oxygenates the water by running it over a series of stones the way water would run in a stream. This improves the water's structure. There's still debate about how this works, but we believe the Vitalizer makes our water extra hydrating. The Vitalizer Plus website says that distilled water is the best water for their product because the spinning in combination with the movement over the stones adds the proper mineralization and makes the water functional. In other words, the water becomes more bioavailable and can be used more readily by the body.

You want to give your body a more alkaline environment because an acidic environment fosters the growth of disease. Given that our atmosphere is highly acidic due to pollution, as are many of the foods we eat (tea, coffee, soda, red meat, processed foods), drinking alkaline water might be a wise health choice. In fact, there is a significant trend toward drinking alkaline water and installing home alkalization systems. From our point of view, that is a little extreme. On the more moderate side, we do drink a 9.5 pH water called Essentia once a week. If your optimum eating and drinking habits aren't yet fully established, it might be a good idea to drink highly alkaline water on a more regular basis as this can offset the amount of acidic foods or drinks you may still be ingesting. Of course, we know that by now you are consuming more and more alkaline foods and beverages every day!

Not all Liquids Are Created Equal

People often think that because they drink a lot of fluids, like coffee, tea and soda, that they're automatically getting their optimal daily intake of water. Not true. While there is plenty of water in coffee, for example, the drink is a diuretic (causes more frequent urination), leaving you less hydrated than you were to begin with. Same story for most teas. Even herbal teas can act as diuretics. And that goes in a huge way for sugary drinks—but of course you're not having those anymore are you?! For pure hydration with nothing negative added like sugar, coloring or empty calories, water is the ticket.

Does Water Have Feelings?

*"In one drop of water are found all the secrets of all the oceans;
in one aspect of You are found all the aspects of existence."*

—KAHLIL GIBRAN

We've been intrigued by the work of Masaru Emoto, a Japanese researcher and author of *The Messages of Water*. Emoto believes that water has a consciousness, an intelligence. He believes that water responds to thoughts and spoken or written words. His books show stunning photographs of frozen water molecules, which he says form differently depending on whether they're exposed to positive thoughts or negative ones. He concludes that happy, harmonious, loving thoughts directed at the water molecules result in a more symmetrical and harmonious structure. Simply writing a message on the side of a bottle of water, he says, changes the nature of the structure. Fascinating idea, isn't it?

Our bodies are made up largely of water, so how do positive and negative thoughts effect our structure? If Emoto is on the right track, then someone who thinks negatively all the time will experience a breakdown on a cellular level. Could it be that a positive person who focuses on the things in life that are going well stands to be a healthier person right down to their body's water molecules?

POINT-EARNING ACTIVITIES CHECKLIST

DRINK PURE WATER

- For one day, every time you instinctively reach for
  coffee, tea or soda, have a glass of water instead.   **10 POINTS**

- Go shopping for a glass water pitcher you like, maybe
  something colorful that inspires you to drink more water.   **5 POINTS**

- Fill a water pitcher, maybe the one you bought in the
  exercise above, with fresh water and add cucumber,
  orange and lemon slices. Enjoy several refreshing
  glasses of this infused water throughout the day.   **10 POINTS**

- After drinking the plastic bottles of water you have
  on hand (and recycling the containers), restock with
  glass bottles from sources you've researched. Think
  local and responsible companies.   **10 POINTS**

- If the price of bottled water is a concern, buy a filter
  for your faucet.   **10 POINTS**

- If you can afford to invest in a filter that covers
  the whole house, go for it. Now your showers
  and baths are healthier. Even the pets you care
  for will be healthier.   **20 POINTS**

- Ask for water without ice every time you go out.
  Ice water lowers your immune system.   **5 POINTS**

- Toss the sodas!   **10 POINTS**

- Try different mineral waters that are naturally sparkling.
  Find water brands that you really enjoy.   **5 POINTS**

TOTAL POINTS _____

CHAPTER 7

CLEANSE AND HEAL

"When 'I' is replaced by 'we,' even illness becomes wellness."

—ANONYMOUS

To be radiantly healthy, we must always look within, or we will always be without. Health always begins from the inside and radiates out! Physical, mental and emotional cleansing—letting go of the old and bringing in the new—is an important key to gaining and maintaining the kind of inner health that results in an outward glow. It is called DETOXIFICATION. When you flush away those internal impurities and toxins, you free yourself body and mind to become authentically YOU. We will help you create a system of detoxification that works for your body.

Detoxification can include anything from drinking distilled water, to fasting, to oral hygiene, to the occasional serious cleanout—a colonic. The purpose of any internal cleansing is mainly to aid your digestion, lymphatic systems and organs to keep them working at optimum performance. When all these systems are working well and we are breaking our food down properly, we absorb nutrients efficiently, eliminate regularly and strengthen our immune system. Seventy percent of the body's cleansing happens through the breath! Twenty percent happens through perspiration, eight percent through urine, and two percent through excrement. Learn to breathe deeply of the healing air around you. Commit to move your body. Replenish your body with pure, clean water. Eat clean, wholesome food. Laugh and look for good in yourself and others. Be happy. Be grateful. This is Nature's way to detox every day.

Helping Our Bodies Detox

Our bodies aren't capable on their own of getting rid of the toxins that bombard them every single day. We have to help them detoxify by getting away from the impure foods and drinks that are causing imbalance. If we allow the toxins to remain and proliferate, the result is inevitable—we get sick. The more we detoxify, the more we create a healthy environment for our organs and cells and the more we can be in tune with what our bodies need. When we become clean on the inside, we clear the way for our bodies and minds to function at their best.

What we find interesting is that it takes a cleanse of some kind for many people to realize how unhealthy they have been. Living sick has become the new normal for most people. An estimated 60 percent of Americans are on a pharmaceutical drug for a mental, physical or emotional illness. What's normal about that? Nothing.

After a 21-day cleanse (whether it is changing how you eat in the morning, adding lots of water, getting rid of soda or deciding to eat only organic and seasonal), you will be able to free yourself of old habits. And then in a total of just 30 short days, you will be able to create new healthy ways of living. Often people will say to us, "Wow, I never knew how tired or depressed I was until I began to detoxify." A good detoxification can help you discover the kind of energy and sense of well-being that you may not have experienced since you were just a young kid.

Disease-Causing Toxins

Every time you eat or drink,
you are either feeding a disease or fighting it.

Diseases—mental, physical and emotional—are often caused by toxic pollution of one form or another. If you are out of harmony with who and what you really are, at some point your electrical and energetic fields can become warped. Your mental processes may not be quite right. You may be drawn to do, think, absorb and consume things that are not good for you—that harm the physical body along with your emotional framework. It may be incompatible foods that cause the disturbance or too much alcohol or sugar or even interactions with angry people. Anger negates love, and the less love there is, the less overall health you will experience. Fortunately, through cleansing and natural healing, you can rid your body of these harmful toxins.

Mariel: I have a passion for making people aware of health, nutrition and lifestyle as it relates to mental well-being. When I eat unhealthy food, I become mentally challenged and off-kilter. When that happens, I ask myself, what have I been eating that's making me feel cloudy-headed? Have I had any gluten? Because of the way we process grain in this country (with hormones and pesticides), I believe it has become toxic to a lot of people (that is why gluten-free has become a huge business). Have I had too much caffeine? Have I gone to the bathroom regularly? And if not, what is causing me to be blocked? Too much sugar, not enough fiber or maybe pasteurized dairy? Whatever the cause, when my body is toxic, my mind is cluttered. I am more emotional and less able to handle my life in a stable way. When this happens, it is time for some sort of cleanse.

Holistic Medicine Versus Western Medicine

First, we want to make it clear that we believe emergency medical treatment in this country is amazing. Saving lives, bringing people back from trauma and putting them back together is something we do with excellence. What we would like to see improve is the illness to wellness part. Traditional doctors are not required to have any training in nutrition. This makes little sense since the large majority of illnesses that doctors attempt to treat are caused by poor nutrition. And, you guessed it, more often than not, the cure is simply a healthy diet.

A major difference between Western medicine and holistic medicine is that Western medicine focuses on and treats a particular ailing part of the body—the symptom rather than the cause of the symptom. Dr. John McDougall, best-selling author and leading nutrition expert, learned this firsthand. As a freshman in college, John McDougall suffered a stroke. Doctors offered no explanations and never asked about his lifestyle, which included a steady diet of chili dogs and other fast food and little to no physical exercise. McDougall discovered through his own research and experience that when he cleansed his body by eliminating harmful foods, he could achieve better health than he'd ever experienced, even as a kid! Now McDougall's mission is to help restore others to optimum health, and he has seen countless individuals discontinue or lower their medication intake for diabetes, heart disease, high blood pressure and many other illnesses simply through learning healthier ways of eating and living. It is amazing what the body can do for itself when we cleanse it and allow it to heal by enjoying clean, healthy foods.

Holistic medicine addresses the whole person—mind, body and spirit—to create an environment in which disease cannot exist. So, for example, in the case of cancer, Western medicine will attack the tumor(s) but may not take into account what led to its appearance. A holistic approach will attempt to discover and correct the underlying disease process. This requires some detective work to ferret out the emotional/physical/environmental factors that might have contributed to the disease in the first place. Return to health may require changes in diet, defensive measures against pollutants and toxins in your environment, and adjustments to assure peak psychological, spiritual and emotional health. The holistic approach is about achieving balance in every area of your life, not just about masking the symptoms of imbalance.

If you are feeling sick, whether it's a head cold or something much more significant, consider the following: What are your stresses? How are you sleeping? What are you eating? What are you drinking? Are you drinking enough water? How much sugar are you taking in? Is a change of weather putting extra stress on your body? The answers to these questions will help you determine the steps you need to take to regain your health.

All of the things we talk about in this book—eating healthy food, drinking pure water, enjoying the outdoors, paying attention to what's in your environment and in the products you use—are actions we can take to boost the health of our immune systems. Cleansing is another tool that can help you live a more balanced life. We'll talk more about the specifics below.

> *Bobby: In my own research, I have yet to find evidence that any degenerative disease can be cured apart from a real vitamin, mineral or food and nutrition factor that helps the body to do its job and heal. We are self-healing, self-sufficient and self-sustaining. When we make a practice of consulting these doctors—Sun, Air, Water, Exercise, Food and Rest—we stay well. No prescription drug has ever cured a single degenerative disease ever that I know of. Yes, they can alleviate symptoms, but the cause of the disease goes untouched. It's like saying, let's get rid of these firemen— they're here so they must be the cause of the fire. In the same way, getting rid of symptoms won't eliminate the cause of an illness; symptoms are only present as a signal that something is going wrong in the body that needs to be investigated.*

Keep Your Head About You

Sometimes life patterns and mental conditioning lock us into certain ailments and pains; this is the mind-body-spirit connection at work. For example, some alternative healers believe that unresolved anger and frustration get stored in the hips, which can make them tight and painful. You've probably had moments when you were so anxious about something that you felt sick to your stomach. Then when the anxiety-causing event passed, *voila*, your queasiness disappeared. Or maybe you got a splitting headache when circumstances made you feel tense and overwrought. These are obvious manifestations of the mind-body-spirit connection, but there can be more subtle disturbances too, and they are different for each of us. We need to recognize these subtle disturbances and address them in a holistic manner.

If you really believed you deserved better, you would have it.

A big part of healing starts with understanding what's blocking you in your mental/emotional world. This may mean delving into your personal history, where you come from, how your parents brought you up, who influenced you. We all translate our emotions with different physical expressions, so as a rule of thumb, tune into yourself at least once a day. Pay attention to how your body feels and how those physical sensations are connected to your thoughts and emotions. If you're feeling discomfort around anything, acknowledge the issue. If it's chronic, talk to someone about it—a friend, a therapist or a counselor. Chances are, if you don't deal with discomforting feelings, they will deal with you, showing up as sickness of one sort or another.

Perhaps you are blocked because the direction you're taking in life is not your path but rather the path of others. Find out what moves you. Do what you love and love what you do! Become the person you know you are. When you choose to be yourself, you will always choose well. You are the only one like you, and that is a powerful statement.

As we've said before, it is important to honor any and all thoughts and feelings, including those that are negative. Denying negative energies doesn't make them go away. We want to understand and observe them, and then when they've had their 15 minutes, to release them. This clears the way for us to embrace our positive thoughts and emotions.

Bobby: We are creating our lives every moment with our thoughts and with the words we choose to give our best attention to. Here are some powerful words to help create your reality: bold, abundant, free, noble, altruistic, compassionate, original, spontaneous, hopeful, wonderful, strong, evolving, good, beautiful, true. It is our choice to incorporate inspiring words and thoughts into our being.

We all need to be cognizant of the words we use and the intentions behind them, what we say to ourselves, and what we put out into the world. This is why we consciously emphasize the first and last thoughts of the day. The way you wake up in the morning, the thought process that rules your day, and the last reflections before going to sleep will orchestrate how you feel and how you heal. (Go back to Chapter 2, Sleep Well, and reread the sections on nightly and morning rituals.)

Ignore Your Age

We are never too old to become younger.

One way to move toward healing is to ignore the *rules* about aging and let yourself be as young as you feel. It's difficult to open yourself to healing when you feel that you are supposed to be getting less active and experiencing aches and pains because, after all, you're getting older. Age, or better yet, *agelessness,* is a mental outlook. It all depends on your perception. You are as young as you feel. Don't celebrate birthdays with a number. Instead, consider them achievements or anniversaries. The signs associated with aging—dry skin, lines and wrinkles, maybe a little less agility—are often more related to what you eat and drink and what you take in mentally and emotionally than they are to the number of years or days you've been on the planet.

We make a point of directing our thoughts to the idea that we're getting younger, healthier and stronger every day. We know that this makes a huge difference in how we feel, and it's much more empowering than to sit around and think, *This hurts, I don't feel well, or I can't* . . . . Forget the negative programming about aging!

There are some great things about having more experience behind you. For us, we don't sweat the small stuff anymore, and we're enormously grateful for what we have. We've learned to stay mindful, to be in the moment throughout the day, to nurture relationships and to recognize the importance of friends. All our years of experience have taught us that life can be remarkably joyful no matter what's going on around us. Our wisdom gives us more life!

The ABCs of Cleansing

When we talk about cleansing, we're talking about ridding the body—the internal organs, the skin, the mouth—of undesirable substances. If you eat well and get the proper enzymes and proper water, you may not need to do any cleanses, ever. But even when we eat well, we still encounter toxins in other forms—through the pollution, dust and chemicals we come in contact with in our everyday lives. When we ingest too many toxins, our liver gets overworked, and once one organ is out of whack, the others start to be affected as well. That's why we recommend cleansing every once in a while.

The goal of cleansing is to remove toxins that inhibit health and the body's natural ability to heal. With cleansing, we're doing our best to work back toward homeostasis, which is our body's choice, by getting rid of unwanted bacteria, waste products, metals and other chemicals that may be lodged in the internal organs, in the cells and in the tissues. Although the body does a remarkable job of getting rid of toxins on its own, there are some that require an extra shove.

Colonics—also called colon irrigation or hydrotherapy—are essentially enemas with a longer reach and are a standard form of cleansing in the Ayurvedic tradition. We recommend this kind of intense cleanse, with your doctor's approval of course, if you suffer from poor elimination or if you are doing an extended juice fast—anything beyond three days. In our experience, brief periods of fasting can yield tremendous results when the colon is cleansed of waste, enabling the body to use the fasting period as a time to heal.

The colonic cleanse is also a powerful motivator. After a colonic, we feel light and energized by getting rid of excess waste and toxins, and we want to continue to reap the benefits through healthy eating. We don't want to put unhealthy foods into our freshly cleansed system. Most people we know experience this same motivation and typically go on to make healthier eating choices.

Ask an experienced friend or a holistic doctor for a referral to a reputable practice that administers colonics. If you are often constipated, this may be part of a solution, along with correcting your diet and getting plenty of water and exercise. Many people who suffer with IBS (irritable bowel syndrome) have also reported dramatic improvement in symptoms following a colonic cleanse.

Other cleanses can be performed at home and may consist of specially formulated drinks, supplements or powders. Cleanses can be focused on the liver, the kidneys and/or the entire body. One short and very effective liver cleanse is Catie's One-Week Liver and Gallbladder Cleanse Kit. Many whole foods markets also carry a variety of similar cleanses.

Addiction Detox Food Program

A cleansing food program can also be used to help break an addiction— to drugs, alcohol, caffeine and sugar. Keep in mind, though, that detox from drugs and alcohol is more complicated than making new dietary choices and requires outside support and assistance, which goes beyond the scope of this book. Here, we are specifically talking about breaking addictions to caffeine, processed/packaged food and sugar. But we can say with confidence that living a cleaner life by implementing the healthy choices we present here in *Running with Nature* will lay a foundation to help support your goal to break other addictions.

It is believed that a physical addiction is broken in 72 hours but that it takes a minimum of 21 days to break a mental addiction to a substance. Even so, it can take much, much longer to actually get the residues of that substance completely out of the body, and that's where clean eating comes in. This kind of food program is covered in Chapter 5, Eat Wholesome Food. We will repeat the most important things here: Eat only clean, simple, organic food, and cut out all processed, packaged, and fake foods to create a clean environment in your body.

Mariel: When I first gave up coffee, I had an extremely strong caffeine addiction. I was fortunate enough to be working with a really good holistic doctor at the time. He told me that it would take from two to six months for the caffeine that was lodged in my tissues to be released, that the body holds on to everything that is not done moderately. In fact, my skin erupted for several weeks after giving up coffee, a sign that the toxins were releasing

*from my body. I had over-caffeinated for years, so it took a long
time to clean it out of my system. Ugh . . .*

Bobby: *I've never had a cup of coffee! From what I hear, coffee
is a quick energy fix for people who need a pick-me-up. I have
been fortunate to always have a lot of energy, so I never went for
the coffee. But I can tell you I have eaten my share of bad food.
As a kid, I ate everything—cookies, candy, cake, doughnuts,
chips, soda, pizza, beer (our dad gave us sips as kids; I started
drinking at 13 years old and quit at 18 years old), canned food,
fast food, packaged, processed, radiated, and pasteurized food,
including sugar cereal with an added spoonful of sugar on top.
And I wondered why I had headaches after drinking the last bit
of sugared milk at the bottom of the cereal bowl. Plus, I drank
huge amounts of pasteurized milk and ate pasteurized cheese and
butter despite the fact that they never set well with me. Yup, I ate
just about everything. My logic was if the food was created it had
to be good for you. My parents didn't know, so I didn't know. We
ate meat, salads and vegetables, a balanced diet, right? Yeah,
except the quality of the food was not good. I remember my family saying that antibiotics and hormones in the meat made you
stronger and healthier and pesticides in the veggies stopped you
from getting bugs and worms! Are you kidding me?*

*At around 33 years old, my hormones started shutting down.
Fourteen hours of sleep wasn't enough, and I was breaking down
constantly, weak and sick with a virus or a cold and plenty of
aches and pains. My journey to health grew exponentially after I
hit rock bottom and changed how I looked at food and health.
After overhauling my diet, I could breathe out of my nose for the
first time ever, felt younger, read more, had more comprehension,
gained more strength and endurance, and began to grow and
expand on every level—body, mind and spirit! Still growing as I
write!*

*Through our different paths, Mariel and I have come to make
some healthy choices that have changed our lives. We eat a lot of
raw food, including some raw meat, dairy, vegetables, honey, eggs
and especially raw fat. Our food is as much as possible farm-to-*

table food. Though our diet consists of a lot of raw foods, we also eat cooked, live, fermented and sprouted food. We know where all of it comes from. We choose range-free, hormone- and antibiotic-free grass-fed meat and healthy raw dairy from goats, cows and sheep that are treated extremely well—Amish food. We have our own chickens and eggs. We eat only organic free-range chickens. We also grow our own fruits and veggies (in two-year cultivated soil), and we buy local organic and biodynamic produce as well. We stock our pantry with organic nuts and seeds and gluten-free bread. We juice, fast, cleanse, take digestive enzymes and eat fermented foods and natural minerals from the ocean and the earth. We take ingestible clay food-based vitamins, Chinese herbs and teas, and rainforest grown herbs and teas. Our spice rack is filled with organic herbs and spices. We use a clean water filtration system that filters our entire house. And of course the five best doctors we visit are Dr. Sun, Dr. Air, Dr. Water, Dr. Exercise and Dr. Nutrition.

Fasting to Cleanse the Body

> *"The best of all medicines is resting and fasting."*
>
> —BEN FRANKLIN

Fasting is a method of cleansing during which you abstain from eating food for short periods of time. A fast can be as short as not eating until lunch or dinner, or it can mean taking a few days drinking only green juices (see our favorites below) and water. We're not suggesting going crazy with this idea—it's just about giving your digestive system a little R & R. And, of course, always check with your naturopathic doctor before embarking on a fast of any kind or any length. We can only tell you what works for us, and because everyone is different, you need to determine what is right for you with supervision from a healthcare specialist.

Cleansing once a week, once a month, biannually or whatever

works best for you is an extremely powerful way of keeping your body toxin free and in homeostasis. In deciding the duration of your fast (several hours, a day, a week or more), the first consideration is your current health. Do you have any conditions or illnesses that would preclude you from fasting? For example, people with blood sugar problems should probably not attempt a full water-only fast. If you are unsure, consult your healthcare professional. You may discover that a few hours of fasting would be fine for you, while a lengthier fast may present a health risk. Also, consider the demands that will be placed on your body at work and at home, and consider your ability to support yourself with rest.

You will also need to decide what type of fast you will do. If you choose a water fast—ingesting nothing but pure water—proceed carefully and really listen to your body to make sure it's benefitting and not being taxed. You may choose to fast with green juice or with water mixed with fresh fruit juice. Organic apple or fresh pineapple juice with ginger is *great* for healing your digestion.

Remember, your fast is personal to you. We are simply giving suggestions based on what works for us. You may want to do your own research on fasting to get an idea of the various options.

Fasting will quickly help you feel more connected with yourself. One of the reasons we think a lot of spiritual teachers and religious groups fast during the year is to heighten their sense of awareness and mental clarity. While fasting, you can temporarily stop and clear out so much of the "noise" that comes from eating too much of anything, especially sugary and caffeinated foods and drinks. The energy normally directed toward digestion can be turned toward a sharper sense of awareness and self *in-tune-ness*. This is why a good time to meditate is before you eat in the morning or before you eat anything heavy. When you're looking for clarity or need your body to focus its energy on healing, it may be helpful to take a responsible break from digestion. Fasting can be the greatest catalyst for your inner physician.

Mariel: I used to fast a lot, but I did it for the wrong reasons. I was doing it because I was modeling or acting and worried about my weight, as opposed to doing it for health reasons. I do believe it is a great idea to give your body a break from digesting food, even for short periods of time. Because of my history with yoyo dieting/fasting and how it messes with my head, I don't do long fasts.

What I like to do is get up early and have my water, then my green tea, and then a small green smoothie (recipe in Chapter 5). I go to a yoga class or take a long hike, and then by 12:30 or 1:00 p.m., I am ready for lunch. Strangely enough, I am not starving— just in need of some fuel, so I eat mostly raw foods that I can digest easily, which still gives my system a break. By evening (no later than 6 p.m. most days in a perfect world when not socializing), I eat a large meal—fish or organic free-range chicken or buffalo with a salad and steamed, sautéed, or roasted veggies. Then I'll have fruit and maybe half a cup of raw yogurt with raw honey before I sleep. I eat a LOT for dinner, and my body is given a break basically 'til dinner the next day. I do this a couple of days a week, and then there are some days where I just need more food during the day.

Sunday is our fun day, so that is the day we have a large breakfast/brunch—gluten-free pancakes or waffles and eggs, etc. This system gives my body the time and space to put its energy into its natural cleansing and healing activities instead of digesting food.

Bobby: *Much simpler than a pure-water fast is a cleanse using green juice and herbal teas. This will give you the nutrition you need while giving your system a break. For somebody like me who loses between five and ten pounds in my sleep, it's very hard to fast. I'll lose extreme amounts of weight quickly if I stop eating. I am a fast metabolizer. But I've noticed that when I take a break using green juice with superfood greens added to it and/or certain enzyme-rich fruits (pineapple, papaya and antioxidant-rich berries) in a blend, I'll lose just a little bit of weight and still feel great. For me, this is a much safer way to fast.*

Mariel and I agree that water-only cleanses are very difficult and somewhat destabilizing. We believe that everybody—every body—is different, so everybody must find out what work best for

*them. We naturally fast while we sleep, and most days I continue
my fast after waking with water, green juice and shakes until I am
hungry for solid food. Eating a healthy diet allows us to cleanse
properly every day.*

How We Fast

For our fasting intervals, which can last from just a few hours to a
day or two, we usually drink green juice—celery, spinach, cucumber
and parsley. Sometimes we'll add a bit of apple later in the day. We
keep our sugar intake low when we fast to reduce work for the pancreas. It's important to stay hydrated, so we make sure to have plenty
of water on hand.

We find that raw, organic apple cider vinegar is also great for
cleansing. We like Braggs Organic Apple Cider Vinegar. We mix 2
tablespoons of vinegar with 1–2 teaspoons of raw, unheated and
untreated honey and 4 ounces of warm water. This is a great way to
clean the digestive tract, and it's also an alkalizing drink, which is
great first thing in the morning. People think that apple cider vinegar
is acidic, but it's actually alkalizing to the body. Same with lemons;
they are acidic outside the body and turn alkaline inside your body.
Both are excellent for cleansing. Lemon and warm water is one of the
simplest morning liver cleanses and one you can do as often as you
like. It is not extreme, and it also helps if you are weaning off high
doses of caffeine. It's a great way to start your day!

We usually juice fast for one week, twice a year. It is nice to fast
during the spring and fall in preparation for the change in temperatures and for foods that will be available during the upcoming season.
Fasts are also helpful during sickness or when improper food has been
eaten. We believe that the body likes breaks from strict regimens. Fasts
are an effective way to give the body a break from constant heavy-
duty digestion and help it to regulate itself.

*Bobby: A friend of ours went on a four-month diet/cleanse to lose
a LOT of weight. He ate clean protein, vegetables and fruit, no
fat and no carbohydrates, and drank plenty of water. He reached*

his weight-loss goal and won a GOLD's Gym competition. But the day he broke his cleanse, he went straight to a couple of fast food places to celebrate. The next morning, he called us from his bed in excruciating pain. He couldn't move. The onslaught of toxins after having eaten such an extremely clean diet for four months literally poisoned his body. He ended up dehydrated, his kidneys shut down, and he had to go to the hospital for saline intravenous treatments. The doctors told him he was very fortunate that the outcome wasn't worse.

When you have completed your fast, be sure to break it healthfully because the body is in a pure and neutral state. Keep hydrated with plenty of good water, and start off slowly food-wise with lightly steamed veggies or vegetable puree and soup. Avoid breads and pastas or any processed or excessively acidic food and drinks. You want to ease your body back into the process of digesting the foods you would normally eat—which by now are clean and healthy!

Oral Hygiene and Holistic Dentists

Good oral care can add years to your life! The mouth contains bacteria that is constantly at work. The waste products that it produces become plaque. Of course, you probably already knew this. But what you may not know is that keeping your mouth clean from that plaque through brushing and flossing may help your heart too. According to the American Academy of Periodontology, people with periodontal disease are almost twice as likely to have coronary artery disease (also called heart disease). On the flipside, Dr. Michael Roizen, author of *Real Age,* says that flossing can *add* six years to your life! Regular flossing helps minimize the amount of bacteria that moves from the mouth to the bloodstream, causing swelling of the arteries and a buildup of arterial plaque.

And the heart isn't the only thing that can be negatively affected by poor dental health. Bacteria that invade the body through the gums have also been linked to an increased incidence of diabetes. The theory is that the bacteria cause an increase in the inflammatory response of the body, which affects insulin receptors. Eventually the pancreas, which secretes insulin, becomes damaged and type-2 diabetes sets in. Premature births and chronic inflammatory conditions have also been linked to poor oral health.

Good dental care is also important because our teeth are connected to specific parts of the body and to different organs. It's all inter-related. An experienced dentist can assess your overall health and wellness by reviewing your dental condition. Presence of disease in a particular part of the body correlates with a specific tooth. Each tooth has a related meridian or "energy highway." An unhealthy tooth con-nected to a weak internal organ can make that organ more problem-atic. When a tooth is in trouble, the energy highway connecting it to its corresponding organ or area of the body is interrupted, and illness occurs or is exacerbated.

No discussion of good dental care would be complete without a word of warning: If you have mercury fillings, get them out of your mouth. Mercury is poisonous. Talk to your dentist about replacing any mercury fillings with porcelain amalgam, and make sure they have experience removing mercury fillings. This needs to be done safely to avoid further exposure.

The good news is that with simple, proper care, your teeth and gums can remain healthy. Here is our oral hygiene regimen: First thing upon awakening, we brush with a thick, wide brush (we like the Radius toothbrush). From time to time, we will dip it in diluted hydro-gen peroxide. We brush our teeth and tongue, then use a tongue scraper followed by a good flossing with Desert Essence tea tree oil dental tape. After all of this fun, we use an electric toothbrush (Oral-B is good) with Tom's natural peppermint toothpaste. Once in a while we use a baking soda tooth powder like Ecodent. We then use a gum stimulator around every tooth, stimulating the gum line.

We recommend holistic dentists who are likely to suggest dietary and lifestyle changes to better support general health as well as give oral/dental care. They may inquire about your mental/physical/spiri-tual well-being and talk about techniques such as yoga, meditation or chakra alignment to further improve the body's relationship with the mouth and teeth. In short, a holistic dentist will examine the whole patient, including his or her emotional attachments, physical health, jaw alignment, diet and lifestyle before deciding upon a treatment plan. Another benefit of seeing a holistic dentist is that they will likely be more conscious about the use of x-rays and will use healthy mouthwashes and cleansers so you aren't ingesting fake sweeteners or synthetic chemicals.

Cleaning Nasal Passages

Neti pots, which look like small porcelain teapots, are used to irrigate the nasal passages in Ayurvedic medicine. A solution of warm distilled water and a small amount of salt—about 1/8 teaspoon for an average neti pot—is poured in one nostril and allowed to flow out the other. (Do this over the sink, tilting the head at about a 45-degree angle so the water can get into one nostril and drain out the other.) You need to use healthy salt such as sea salt or a fine salt that the neti pot makers recommend to make the water solution. This becomes a powerful cleanser. If you have sinus blockage, this can be a gentle but effective way to get things moving again. Use of a neti pot can also help with allergies, nasal dryness and congestion. You can get a neti pot at many yoga studios, natural grocery stores or on amazon.com.

> *Bobby: We both feel that the greatest neti pot of all is the ocean! While we're getting turned about in the waves, the salt water cleans out all debris from our sinuses. Plus, we're left feeling energized, refreshed and restored.*

> *Mariel: Yes, the ocean is fantastic, but it's not always possible or practical. I find that if I start to get a cold, cleansing with a neti pot quickly clears up my cold symptoms like sore throat and stuffy nose. During high cold season, or during a change of season, if I use a neti pot every day, I typically don't get sick.*

Cleansing Your Environment

Along with a healthy body, we think it's imperative to have a clean and uncluttered environment. Too much stuff is distracting on every level—from the visual to the energetic. Clearing away all the extraneous things in your life is a powerful form of cleansing and can have a powerful effect on your overall outlook.

Material objects have energy. We interact with everything in our lives on an energetic level. If you have more stuff than you need, that stuff is actually draining your energy. If you are surrounded by clutter, your energy is being sapped by it, probably without your even realizing it.

We're a country of bumper stickers that read, "He who dies with the most toys wins." Our "stuff" symbolizes our status. As a result, we've become a nation of consumers and pack rats. We really believe we need all our stuff. We think it brings us happiness and security. But, in truth, it doesn't. As soon as you buy the one thing you absolutely *must have,* another thing pops up demanding possession with the same unwarranted urgency.

We're not advocating abandoning your life or giving up all your things and becoming homeless. But everyone can benefit from de-cluttering and simplifying. It will free up a tremendous amount of life energy. If you were to reduce your life to only the bare necessities—one frying pan instead of three, a few good pens instead of a dozen throwaways, the clothes you actually wear rather than the ones that have been in the closet untouched for years—you might be astounded by how little you actually need to be happy and healthy. In our society, we think our worth is derived from our things. Ironically, by losing them, we gain a better relationship with ourselves. And that relationship leads to a better understanding and acceptance of who we really are. It's so freeing to release the burden of the things that insulate us.

When life is simplified, it's easier to organize, and when life is organized, chaos has no place to live. Just think about the time you've wasted trying to find keys or a wallet or glasses that weren't where they were supposed to be or were lost in a mess of clutter.

Pick a day to go through the closets or cabinets of a single room in your home and de-clutter. When in doubt, ask yourself when you last used the item in question and why you need it. Answer honestly! If you really can't let go, put a "use by" date on it, say, two weeks. If in two weeks time you still haven't used this thing, face the fact: you don't need it!

Give it away, take it to Goodwill or another charity, or toss it if it is no longer useful. If you've got stacks of CDs, put the music on your computer or iPod. Scan important documents and store them electronically to clear some of the clutter from your file cabinet. And while we're talking about paper clutter, think about switching to online billing or automatic bill payments. There are so many ways to simplify your environment when you take some time to think about it.

Bobby: Some of my happiest times in life occurred when I had virtually no possessions, no home, no job, no agenda. I've lived in my truck with nothing more to my name than a cell phone, and sometimes the cell would be down for quite some time. I would make calls from pay phones. My only financial obligations were feeding myself, paying a small phone bill and putting gas in my truck to take me on my next adventure. I have traveled back and forth across the country some 87 times. Several times I was hauling camera equipment and getting paid to see the entire country. I stopped at national parks, beaches, mountains and deserts. It was heaven on earth. Without all the responsibilities of maintaining material things, I experienced a true freedom that most people have not felt since they were kids. And I had the perspective of an adult to appreciate it.

Take Responsibility for Your Healing

Now that we've gotten the cleansing regimens in place, our bodies have the foundation for healing. We believe that healing is our responsibility—we have to treat our bodies well with the right nutrition and the right emotional and spiritual setting in which to thrive. This book is intended to help you to adjust your lifestyle to create optimum health. Transferring your power to doctors and others without question when you are ill is, in our opinion, irresponsible. You can gather tons of help, advice and a diagnosis from the medical profession, but ultimately no one knows your body better than you. You are your own best advocate, and when you learn to listen to your body's messages, you're that much better suited for the task. Your attitude toward your personal healing is essential to creating perfect health for YOU.

Benefits of Hydrotherapy

Cold water stimulates your body. It turns your system on. During the hot months here in Los Angeles, we love jumping into the ocean for a cold plunge a couple of times a day. When we go to the mountains, we take our dips in the icy rivers. The energy we feel after being in a cold lake or waterfall is amazing. But you don't have to live near a cold body of water to get these benefits. A shower will suffice. Even something as simple as a shower, bath or whirlpool is considered hydrotherapy. If you alternate from hot to cold water, it's especially stimulating—spas often have cold plunge pools next to the warm whirlpools, and Nordic traditions include running from a hot sauna out into the snow or a frigid lake. That freezing dip is also a helpful remedy for depression—almost a shock treatment of sorts, but a lot kinder and more enjoyable.

Heat causes your muscles to expand; cold makes your blood vessels contract. So the blood speeds up and slows down, speeds up and slows down, and so on. This creates a tremendous movement of blood throughout your system. Bringing blood to specific areas of the body heals those areas and benefits the body as a whole. This is an energizing, invigorating and healing therapy accessible to everyone.

You can also try the hot-cold combo after exercising. Alternating hot and cold in the shower will move the lactic acid out, get your blood going and strengthen your immune system. If you have an injury, the blood flowing through the injured area can accelerate healing. Physical therapists typically recommend heat for chronic injuries to help loosen up the muscles and tissues and cold for acute injuries to reduce swelling. We have found benefits from the combination of the two.

Bobby: Cold water invigorates you at every level. Simply jump in and wake up! I jump into rivers, lakes, ponds and oceans. Our own pool is 41 degrees in the middle of the winter, and we jump in nearly every day. Try it for yourself, even if all you have available to you is a cold shower. It boosts your energy and your immune system, gets your blood pumping, burns calories, keeps your skin and hair healthy and increases testosterone.

Mariel: *Cold awakens your senses—stimulates your brain to think more clearly. Comedians often keep their studios at 55°F because it makes them sharper. When I've gone on* The David Letterman Show, *I've almost frozen to death.*

Natural Skin and Body Care Products

In Chapter 5, the food chapter, we talked about processed, chemicalized "dead" foods. Many skin and body care products also fall into the dead category. The skin is the body's largest organ, and it is porous. If you wouldn't eat or drink something, think twice about putting it on your skin where it will be absorbed into your body. If you can't pronounce the ingredients in your oil or lotion, or if you don't know what an ingredient is, do a little research before you slather it on.

The skin needs to be cleaned, moisturized and occasionally scrubbed to maintain its healthy condition. We use NaPCA spray on our face to keep our skin moisturized. (Several companies make these sprays including Nu Skin and Twinlab.) NaPCA is a naturally occurring compound in the body responsible for moisturizing the skin. NaPCA sprays work by pulling water from the air into the skin, so it is really hydrating. This is a way of preventing dry skin rather than just covering it up. Sometimes we make body moisturizer from coconut oil and ginger together, and we've also made a great conditioner out of an egg and avocado mixture.

Bobby: *To protect my skin, I wear a rash guard (the one I wear for surfing under my wetsuit) when I go out hiking, biking or otherwise spend hours in the sun. When I'm climbing, I put that on because I know I am getting a sunblock of 50 without chemicals,* *and it protects the whole body up to the bottom of the chin. Because I spend so much time in the sun—I'm sometimes outside all day long—I make sure I'm covered up, especially during midday. None of us wants to age prematurely, and overexposure causes sun damage, which in turn leads to aging. Morning sun and late day sun for me.*

As we discussed in Chapter 1, for the most part, sunscreens should be natural with no chemical ingredients. Titanium dioxide and zinc oxide are highly effective natural mineral sunblocks that lie on top of the skin rather than being absorbed. We have also rubbed on peanut oil, which has natural sun-protection properties, the night before going out in the sun. However, peanut oil only blocks about 20 percent of the sun's UV rays, so if you tend to burn or will be out in the sun for a long time, stick to the higher SPF sunblocks. Another effective natural sunscreen is Bayleaf extract spray . . . it prevents a burn naturally. And don't forget about covering up. Wear a hat or long sleeves if you plan on spending a prolonged amount of time out in the sun.

> *Mariel: The skin is the largest organ in the body, and it absorbs nearly everything. So natural skin care is incredibly important. Natural skin care promotes a vibrancy that you just don't get when you use chemicals on your skin. The most important thing to look for in skin care products is that they are free of parabens, polymers and alcohol. You don't want to be absorbing petrochemicals (chemicals derived from petroleum that are commonly found in skincare products), and alcohol is drying.*

Many natural products also contain essential oils, which provide other healing benefits. The natural scents can have a variety of different effects—from stimulating to calming. Shopping for skin care products is personal. Go to the store and smell different products to see what you like, test them to see what they do on your skin, and of course read the labels to make sure they don't contain dyes and chemicals. Think of your skin care regimen as an extension of your diet. Become conscious of what's in it.

Essential Oils

Records dating back to 4,500 B.C. refer to essential oils, some of the most powerful therapeutic agents known. They have been used throughout history for healing a wide variety of health complaints, including nervousness, fever and infections of the skin and throat. With the advance of antibiotics and prescription drugs in the twentieth century, the therapeutic use of essential oils was overlooked. During the last decade, they have been steadily reclaiming their popularity.

In their pure state, essential oils can be up to 10,000 times more concentrated than the plants from which they're extracted. Uplifting, protective, calming and/or regenerating, these distilled oils, often referred to as the "life blood" or "essential essence" of a plant, come from shrubs, flowers, trees, roots, bushes and seeds. They not only determine the plant's aroma but are also vital for its growth and survival. These same vital qualities work in us to heal the mind, body and spirit.

Essential oils can be inhaled directly from the bottle, diffused into the air using a cold-mist essential oil diffuser and directly applied behind the ears, over vital organs, to the feet or to other areas as needed for a specific treatment. (Dilution with a blending, or carrier, oil such as jojoba, olive, grape seed or vitamin E is recommended.) The oils can also be consumed, a few drops placed on the tongue, or added to water or another beverage. Some people place several drops into an empty vegetable capsule and swallow it that way. Be careful to ingest only therapeutic-grade, GRAS (generally regarded as safe for consumption by the FDA) essential oils. The following are some common ailments and symptoms and the essential oils used to treat them:

♦ **To boost alertness, concentration, and recall:** Diffuse peppermint oil in the room while studying to improve concentration and accuracy. Inhale peppermint oil while taking a test to improve recall.

♦ **For anxiety:** Apply topically and inhale oils of lavender, geranium or chamomile.

♦ **As an appetite suppressant:** Inhale the fragrance of peppermint oil.

- **For coughs and allergies:** Apply oils of lavender, chamomile, eucalyptus, peppermint, ravensara, lemon, thyme or angelica topically.

- **For calming and as a sleep aid:** Diffuse oils of lavender, orange, bergamot, geranium or chamomile and apply to the spine and feet before bedtime to aid relaxation.

- **For detoxing liver and gallbladder:** Apply oils of cardamom, geranium, chamomile or blue tansy to bottom of feet.

- **To detox kidneys:** Apply oils of juniper or fennel to bottom of feet.

- **For dry skin or scalp:** Mix lavender oil with blending vegetable oil; apply to skin and massage into the scalp.

- **As an exercise enhancement:** Drink a few drops of peppermint oil in water before and during a workout to boost your energy and reduce fatigue.

- **For a fever:** Apply oils of peppermint, lavender and lemon to the feet and calves.

- **As first aid:** Apply lavender oil on minor cuts and scrapes to help stop bleeding and disinfect the wound.

- **To freshen breath:** Place a drop of peppermint or spearmint oil on the tongue.

- **For tooth pain or bleeding gums:** Rub a drop or two of clove oil blended with vegetable oil on gums.

- **For headache:** Apply peppermint oil on the temples and on the back of the neck and inhale deeply.

- **For hiccups:** Apply a drop of peppermint oil on each side of the fifth cervical vertebra (up three notches from the large vertebra at the base of the neck).

- **For immune support:** Apply a few drops of oregano, cinnamon, frankincense, thyme, clove or cumin blended with vegetable oil to spine or bottoms of feet.

- **For insect bites:** Apply oils of lavender, Roman or German chamomile, Idaho tansy or eucalyptus topically on insect bites to reduce itching and swelling.

- **As an insect repellant:** Mix several drops of the following oils with water and apply topically: lavender, citronella, peppermint, eucalyptus and lemongrass.

- **For minor burns and sunburn:** Apply lavender oil on a minor burn or sunburn to decrease pain and reduce swelling.

- **For mood elevation:** Diffuse or inhale lemon or peppermint oil.

- **For nosebleed:** Put a drop of lavender oil on a tissue and wrap it around a small chip of ice. Push the tissue-covered ice chip up under the middle of the top lip to the base of the nose and hold as long as comfortable or until the bleeding stops (do not freeze the lip or gum).

- **For nausea, heartburn, indigestion, flatulence and diarrhea:** Apply oils of peppermint and chamomile to the stomach. May also ingest as a tea with warm water.

- **For PMS and menopausal symptoms:** Apply oils of clary sage, anise, fennel, geranium or bergamot to the abdomen and lower back.

- **For sore muscles, joint stiffness, inflammation and bruising:** Mix essential oils of peppermint, Idaho balsam fir, wintergreen or birch with a blending oil and apply topically.

Bee Pollen for Allergies

Bee pollen contains 22 amino acids and is made up of about 40 percent protein. If you suffer from a pollen allergy (aka hay fever), one natural remedy is to take bee pollen supplements that are derived from bees. Visit your local farmers market and see if there's a honey maker who can supply you with local bee pollen. Ingesting the bee pollen helps the body build up an immunity to that pollen, thereby reducing allergy-related symptoms. Be careful using this remedy—first take only a small granule as a test to make sure that you don't have an adverse reaction. You can also eat raw, untreated local honey, which may help relieve allergies as well.

Being Your Authentic Self Creates Healing

Being true to yourself, living as your authentic Self, makes you a happier person. It also helps you to heal by stimulating your immune system. Your whole being becomes activated on all the levels it should be activated on, and the places that have been shut down or shut off in your body and mind get recharged. By paying attention to your body's cleanliness, inside and out, by listening to signs of dis-ease and helping to fortify those areas, you're giving yourself a leg up in every aspect of your life. Simply by getting out in Nature and inviting more natural things into your body, you're activating your body's innate ability to repair itself.

Every choice we make has a consequence, even if we don't always see them immediately. When we begin to choose more consciously, we see the results in our health, in our appearance and in our emotional well-being. We connect to who we really are.

We've given you a lot of information in these chapters so far. It may seem overwhelming, but we promise that as you start incorporating these ideas into your daily life, and as you begin to see and feel the results, they will become second nature. You won't even recognize that earlier, duller, disconnected Self. Keep with it!

POINT-EARNING ACTIVITIES CHECKLIST

CLEANSE AND HEAL

- Spend a few minutes when you first wake up assessing your mood. Before you get out of bed, see if you can find any areas of anxiety. Just notice. **10 POINTS**

- One or two days a week (at least), calculate how you feel emotionally. Write it down. Then check in physically. Do you feel unwell in any way—aches, muscle tension, stomach upset? See if any patterns emerge relating to your health and your emotions. **10 POINTS**

- Pick a day to fast until lunch, keeping yourself hydrated with green juices and/or plenty of water. If that goes easily, maybe you can fast until dinner. **10 POINTS**

- Pay attention to your youth, not your age. The next time you're tempted to say, "I'm too old to do _____" rethink that thought. How about, "I'd love to try_____!" Or if the activity really is out of your physical realm, maybe there's a happy modification: "I think I'll pass on the sky dive, but I'd love to go up in the plane with you!" **10 POINTS**

- Choose a room in your home and spend an hour or two de-cluttering it. (If your rooms are too over-whelming, start with your desk or bureau.) If a couple of hours doesn't make a dent, set aside a day and finish the job! **10 POINTS**

- The next time you see your dentist, ask him or her to check your mouth for mercury fillings. If you have any, have them replaced. Make sure the dentist you use knows how to remove mercury fillings safely. **10 POINTS**

- Try the hot/cold dynamic in the shower—spend 20 seconds under the hot water, then switch to cold and stay under for another 20 seconds. Go back and forth up to seven times and notice how your body responds.   **10 POINTS**

- The next time you have the opportunity at a gym or spa, don't just sweat it out in the steam room or sauna—take the plunge! Hop into the cold pool or into a cold shower.   **10 POINTS**

- Check your lotions and sunscreens to see what's in them. If the ingredients sound like chemicals, they probably are. Replace those products with natural alternatives.   **10 POINTS**

- Go to your health food or naturopathic store and invest in some essential oils to use as home remedies. Peppermint (good for energy and digestion) and lavender (calming and good for skin) are especially versatile—start with them. Or ask the salesperson to help you choose something that addresses a current health concern.   **10 POINTS**

TOTAL POINTS _____

CHAPTER 8

LAUGH AND PLAY

"You don't stop laughing because you grow old.
You grow old because you stop laughing."

—MICHAEL PRITCHARD

Think about your summers as a kid and how time didn't exist . . . days were long and full and you had to be dragged out of your tree fort or off your bike to come inside for dinner. You ate as fast as you could so you didn't lose a moment of the fun you were having with your friends playing games or building the perfect bike or skateboard ramp. Every moment was focused on doing the important things you needed to do—exercise your imagination and be right where you were in the moment. Laughing, creating, dreaming, playing . . . that's how we grew up.

Who says you have to give that up just because you're an adult? Who says that because you have a job and children of your own you have to give up being a kid yourself? You can play and become whimsical again. If you plan it right, it won't take away from your responsibilities as a father, mother, employee or spouse. Instead, it will simply add to your happiness account and help you be more present in all the other areas of your life.

Play is the biggest step to becoming the true, youthful YOU. Give yourself one hour a day, that's just 4 percent of the day, to PLAY. The more we laugh and play, the happier we become, and the more connected we are to one another and to ourselves. Rediscover your passion for fun and you'll feel younger and more alive!

The two of us really connect in our desire to not grow up. We believe that we are not meant to slow down because we are 50. We believe we are meant to get better and healthier, and every day we make that choice. We choose to continue to experience the adventure of life with a child's open imaginative mind, to live in the moment, to laugh spontaneously and to be as silly as we can. Remember, being silly is a way of life, and being serious is something temporary that you have to do until you get to be silly again.

We act like kids together throughout the day. Sometimes we are seven years old. Other times we are teenagers. As far as physical activity level is concerned, we pretty much remain in our twenties. We are wise *young* folks. Our ability to laugh and play is a major part of why we look and feel so young. It's a key to our happiness.

We are not asking you to shirk your responsibilities as an adult; we are recommending you relearn how to approach your life. You can start by consciously choosing the thoughts, attitudes, beliefs and actions that bring you happiness and make you laugh like when you were young.

In their book *Self Empowerment—Nine Things the 19th Century Can Teach Us About Living in the 21st,* B. Anne Gehman and Ellen Ratner discuss the teachings of James Freeman Clarke, 19th century orator and preacher. Clarke believed that in order to live well and fully, every individual must develop certain areas of his or her life. Interestingly, along with such areas as education, use of time, and intuitive powers, Clarke also lists "amusement and play." He states, "The love of play and sport shows that amusement is evidently one of the original instincts of human nature . . . Intense enjoyment of play enables children to support pain, teaches them to obey rules, to control themselves, to submit to discipline, to bear fatigue without complaint, and so largely helps in the formation of character." Clarke recognized also that taking the time to play brings us back to a place of freshness in mind and heart. We are better able to move back into work and do it well when we have given ourselves fully to the recreational (truly re-creational) aspects of our lives.

Reactivating your playful child Self takes some dedication. It's easy to let life's responsibilities curb what might have once been a wide-eyed enthusiasm for new adventures, unselfconscious creativity, sheer goofiness. Most of us have less time to engage in hobbies and sports as our lives become more complicated, and a lot of our daily routine involves watching a clock to be sure we're beginning and ending our pursuits on schedule. Time to shift that focus.

Play Games

> *"You can discover more about a person in an hour of play than in a year of conversation."*
>
> —PLATO

We often look to Nature to reconnect with our authentic Selves and spring into the child mind. We actually play games like tag, hide-and-seek, leap frog, wiffle ball and slackline challenges. We're not kidding! You'd be amazed at the joy and exhilaration these games bring out in us, not to mention the fact that healing endorphins (feel-good brain chemicals) are released during play. Play games, especially physical ones, because they break the monotony of being a serious adult, they shift energy, and they help create a new outlook on life no matter what's going on. Why should we deprive ourselves of simple joys that are so much a part of who we are (or were) and are so easily accessible?

We do the absolute silliest things—and we're not embarrassed to share them. We sing in the car at the top of our lungs, making up new words to old songs—sometimes because we never knew the correct lyrics. This alone can send us into a tailspin of hysterical laughter, and we'll actually have to pull the car over because we're laughing so hard. These experiences of pure joy are among the most meaningful restorative moments we have.

Mariel: Even though my nature is funny, my childhood was particularly chaotic and devoid of laughter. My 24-year marriage lacked it as well. In fact, one of my greatest embarrassments today is how extremely difficult it was for me to laugh and play with my kids as they were growing up. I just couldn't seem to let myself do it. I think this is because my parents never had fun with me, so I was never given the model for how to do it with my own kids. I would go out to the park, for example, but it's like I was a big clock. All I could do was keep track of the time. I couldn't let myself relax and play. There was also an element of "I didn't get to have fun as a kid, how come my kids get to?" This is an awkward admission, because it shows how the Little Mariel inside me was never given enough freedom to play and laugh. Oh, how that has changed!

No Time Zone

During our time off, our playtime, we create a sense of timelessness. Watches, dates and days of the week have no functional status. We probably experience this most when rock climbing. You have to be so focused on what you're doing in order not to fall that you really can't have thoughts about anything else. It's an activity that takes you right out of your head.

Too often as adults, it's easy to feel like you're being moved along the raging river of time, getting older without choice. We would like to encourage you to challenge this perception, to tell yourself instead, "I have the ability today to be as childlike and time-free as I was when I was a kid. I simply have to choose it."

Creating space for You is a conscious choice. It's not selfish; it's essential. You know how airline safety rules insist that you put your own oxygen mask on first before helping those around you in the case of an emergency? Finding time for playfulness is the same thing. If you can't keep your own life in balance, you won't have what it takes to help others. And if you're a parent, you want to give your kids the example of a happy and balanced life so they can lead one too.

Monkey Bars and Road Trips

Think about what you used to do for fun as a child and reenact it. For us, this often means—you guessed it—going outside. We sometimes visit local school playgrounds after hours and swing as high as we can on the swings and hang from the monkey bars and the rings. Sometimes we go for a fun bike ride or play Frisbee. Recently, on a trip to Big Sur, we climbed a giant tree. The branches were all fairly close together, so it was more about the adventure than about a challenge. That made it so much fun. One of the best parts of being a kid was getting to climb trees. It's just as great as an adult.

One prerequisite for enjoying these childhood activities today is to undertake them without an agenda—you're just exploring. Play should be totally free from responsibilities or time restraints. That's part of the power of this gift you are giving yourself. It's never too late to become the child you wish you had been.

For us, road trips are another form of play. We just get in the car and head somewhere for the weekend, for a day, or even a few hours. The time we spend in the car is incredibly fun. The hardest part, of course, is coming back! On our road trips, the car becomes home. We bring along with us everything we might need: food, supplies and clothes for climbing, swimming, sleeping out—almost anything that we may decide to do. We allow ourselves to be spontaneous, stopping as frequently as we like when something catches our interest. In the last chapter, we talked about plunging into cold water as therapy, but even that becomes play for us. We always jump in with a sense of humor, splashing and laughing about how cold it is and how funny we must look.

Even if you can only get out for one day on the weekend, just go out and really choose to be playful, to have fun, to be silly! Don't worry about where you might end up or when you're coming back. Be an explorer, with that passionate curiosity you used to have as a kid. If you don't have a day right now, start small by carving out a little bit of time—a few hours or so.

We all have obligations, between family, work and everything else going on in our lives. Even a small shift toward giving yourself a little playtime can enhance other areas of your life. When we take care of ourselves (and that includes having fun), it serves everyone else in our lives. When we're happier, we treat others better. Giving ourselves that fun time, that gift of happiness, fills us up so that we can be happier around others. Giving others the gift of your happiness is a great way to *pay it forward*. It's contagious and others can't help but join you.

Find the Balance

Who in their right mind ever wants playtime to end? But the reality is that when you give yourself time to play, you don't harbor resentment about the time you need to work. As adults, we want the rewards of a job or career and the material things it affords us, so we need to find peace and contentment within this work/play balance. A healthy life requires balance in all aspects.

Too much play without attention to responsibilities means not much will get done; too much responsibility without enough play is a prescription for a stressed-out, unhappy life. The happy medium? Take care of yourself and those you love while giving yourself permission each day to spend some time acting like a kid, playing and having fun.

We have to show up for what life throws at us and deal with our commitments, but we don't have to let them overwhelm the innate enthusiasm and wonderment we were born with. Once again, we're looking for a real relationship with our authentic Self, and that means excavating the essence of our personality, discovering the keys that make us uniquely ourselves.

Bobby: Constantly being serious leads to a life of confinement. Whether it's a business meeting, an event, a class or any job, for me there is always room for laughter. When I see or feel tension from the seriousness in a room, I just can't help it—I have to start goofing around. Life is too short, I say, so live it with laughter. A quick comment or simple gesture helps change the heavy into light. A couple of years ago, when I was at the movie theater with my family, my mother was being so serious about the movie that

*we were about to see. So I grabbed her and hip tossed her, and
we both went to the ground together. She just started laughing.
People were looking at us like we were absolutely crazy. We
laughed and laughed, and she immediately got out of her "serious" mode.*

Healing Through Laughter

Laughter is a great pattern interrupter. When we're angry, it can
change our mood in a second. It can stop an argument or a fight in
its tracks. Stepping back from the heat of an argument to diffuse it
with a joke requires a lot of awareness and self-discipline (muscles
you've hopefully been cultivating with this book), but if you can har-
ness them in a tense situation, if you can find a shred of absurdity that
might help everyone involved lighten up, you've learned to use an
invaluable tool. Very little gets accomplished when we discuss problems while we're angry.

Laughter is also a proven healer. At Honolulu's Queens Medical
Hospital, a palliative-care nurse who was also a comedian started an
in-house comedy channel. Local comedians donated a lineup of skits.
The hospital found that patients had fewer complaints of discomfort
and asked for less pain medication when they were given access to the
channel. The staff benefitted too, often laughing with their patients
while watching the routines. The shared moments were healing for all
involved.

There's a reason these patients needed less pain medication. Laughter releases endorphins that actually work to block pain receptors.
And the benefits of laughter don't stop there. Researchers at Loma
Linda University's Schools of Allied Health (SAHP) and Medicine say
the body responds to laughter like it responds to moderate exercise
and that laughter can enhance mood, decrease stress hormones,
enhance immune activity, lower bad cholesterol and systolic blood
pressure, and raise good cholesterol (HDL). Cancer Treatment Centers of America even use laughter therapy as part of their program for
healing both patients and their families. Like we've always heard,
laughter *is* the best medicine.

The movie *Patch Adams,* based on the life of Dr. Hunter "Patch" Adams, echoes the message of healing through laughter. The movie beautifully portrays Adams' philosophy that humor and play are essential to physical and mental well-being. Dr. Adams received the Peace Abbey Courage of Conscience Award in 1997 and often travels to other countries where he dons a clown suit in an effort to bring humor to patients, orphans and others while promoting an alternative holistic model of healthcare.

Just Start Smiling

In spiritual circles, there is often talk about initiating a smile. If you can smile, even when you're not inclined to, the very gesture will create an uplifting energy, and then the real smile will come. In other words, "Fake it 'til you make it." Pretty soon, your faking it will turn into a genuine smile that may inspire others to smile too.

If you've been participating in the Point-Earning Activities in this book—if you're eating right and getting exercise, spending time outside, and drinking lots of good water, we bet you'll be smiling and laughing a lot more than you were when you started Chapter 1. When you feel good about yourself, you're happy; when you're happy, you smile; when you're smiling, other happy people gravitate toward you. Laughter ensues!

Even if you're a serious professional who deals with sober issues in an office full of sober people, it's okay—and even more important—to have fun. Put a smile on your face and see if it doesn't bring a positive energy to everyone in your workplace.

> *Bobby: We are led to believe that as adults we have a serious role in society for which we must conduct ourselves a certain way and that there is no room for silliness. But you can have many moments of fun, of laughter, of being kid-like, and still be responsible. You don't have to stop playing or disown that integral part of your nature that keeps you young. Sometimes when people have children of their own they are able to reconnect to this place and give themselves permission to play. However, many people, as Mariel explained earlier, don't allow themselves that opportu-*

nity. It is a choice to be childlike, to think from a child's point of view, to be silly. It's a part of our nature that most are not honoring. So honor it. Be happy!

Let It Go!

Can you give yourself permission to belly laugh once a day? You'll be amazed at the way this shifts your energy. Watch a funny movie, read something uplifting, listen to music, put yourself in a position where you can create laughter with others. And stop hanging around with people who kill your joy! You know the kind—the ones who thrive off the negative energy of being angry or unhappy all the time.

By the way, we understand that changing emotional patterns isn't easy. Sometimes it means having to admit that the way you've been approaching life isn't working. That's not the point though. The good news, and the area where the emphasis belongs, is that you've decided to make a change, to opt for the positive.

One key to maintaining happiness is to give up trying to control the outcome of everything in your life. Being in control and needing to know the end result of all your choices ahead of time is a recipe for disappointment. Your success in anything, even in adopting the ideas in this book, requires you to allow the process to unfold in the right way for you and to trust that it will. How it unfolds may be nothing like you planned. Your joy may come from a crazy adventure like Hula-Hooping or from a silly song you just have to sing alone in your living room or playing hide-and-seek with your partner. Your spirit's needs will reveal themselves as you become more aware of all the choices you are making, from food to morning thoughts to playful action. Live in the present moment—after all, that's all there really is.

Mariel: When I first met Bobby (four years ago) and we began to spend more and more time together, I learned that it was okay to laugh and play. Sounds crazy but I really didn't know that it was all right. I became so much happier—but my children didn't recognize me. It isn't that they didn't want me to be happy, but they were confused by the change in me. It was almost as if they felt betrayed. It took some courage for me to let that be okay and to allow myself to be happier anyway. I knew that in time they would come to understand and trust that the change in me was a positive one. Now my girls and I have laughing fits together, and our communication is completely open. The relationship that has grown from my trusting my own joy allows me to love my girls and appreciate them more than I ever had, and in turn, they see me as I truly am.

Being Happy Takes Commitment

We believe that we are all put on this planet to live, love and laugh—to share our light and joy with others. Being happy is a choice and requires commitment, especially when we first decide to embrace it. But being unhappy requires more physical energy. The old saying is true—it requires more muscles to make a frown than it does a smile. And being unhappy drains us emotionally. What are the negative thoughts that might be bringing you down and blocking you from the freedom to laugh and play? Attempt to recognize them, and then let them go. While we all have moments of feeling down and less than optimistic, harboring and recycling the negative stuff is debilitating. It may seem difficult to do, but just make a commitment to see the negativity that you harbor. See it, welcome it, and say to yourself, "I can let this thought go now." Keep saying that until those thoughts lessen and are no longer there. Doesn't it feel like "a weight has been lifted," as the expression goes? For more ideas on how to deal with negative thoughts, look back at our discussion on meditation in Chapter 4.

You can even use your physicality to make a mental shift toward happiness. If you're stuck in a dark place, go outside and walk around the block. If it's the middle of the night, try doing a few jumping jacks. Change your environment. Take a break with the conscious intention to "shift your energy."

Decide to be happy, make the effort and the rewards will grow with compounded interest. You may find that being happy is your default state of mind. Try it. For today, choose to be a person who laughs and smiles instead of frowns. Give yourself permission to PLAY. Watch how you shift your life attitude.

POINT-EARNING ACTIVITIES CHECKLIST

LAUGH AND PLAY

- When you wake up tomorrow, before you get out of bed, decide to be happy. Smile even if you don't want to—it will shift your mood.   **10 POINTS**

- When the day's first irritation gets to you, remember your decision to be happy. Stick to it, while acknowledging the issue that may have come up.   **10 POINTS**

- Play hide-and-go-seek. Go ahead—it's fun!   **10 POINTS**

- Make fun of yourself. Who are you to be so serious anyway? Allow your energy to shift and find the joy that exists all around, no matter what you think you feel right now. Make a choice to have a child's mind and get over stuff fast!   **10 POINTS**

- Do you have a game you can play with a few friends? Charades is always fun!   **10 POINTS**

- The next time you find yourself in an altercation of some sort, step back and find a way to diffuse the tension with humor.   **10 POINTS**

- Got a Hula-Hoop? Now's the time!   **10 POINTS**

- Belly laugh five times in a day. You can fake the first ones. See if the rest come naturally.   **10 POINTS**

- Smile at the next driver who tries to cut you off.   **5 POINTS**

- Before you sleep tonight, make the commitment to wake up happy, joyous and accepting of how your life unfolds the following day.   **10 POINTS**

TOTAL POINTS _____

CHAPTER 9

ADVENTURE

"Do one thing every day that scares you."

—ELEANOR ROOSEVELT

Adventure is a mindset . . . a lifestyle choice. Doing something that takes you to your edge or scares you just a little activates your brain cells and revitalizes your body. It makes you feel alive. It's time to step outside your comfort zone and propel yourself into the unknown! We're not being metaphorical here—we mean, literally, put the iPad aside and move body parts other than your texting fingers.

One prime adventure for us is going to wild places where few people have gone and reconnecting to the immense power surrounding us. When we venture out and learn a new physical skill or step into a challenging wildlife setting, we step into the present moment. When you step into the NOW, you get closer to who you really are. Do something physically adventurous, something you've never tried before, or at least not lately. If your adventure is climbing or wind surfing . . . great. Go for it! It could be riding a bike on a dirt road and finally one day riding on a trail and calling yourself a mountain biker. The important thing is to get out there and do something that makes your stomach jump a little and makes you grin with accomplishment. Get your body moving! Get off the couch and meet yourself. Find your edge and find YOU!

The Benefits of Adventure

The happiest people don't have the best of everything;
they make the best of everything.

Adventure is not about seeking an adrenaline rush; it's about facing a challenge and then enjoying the absolute calm and peace that result from the action. Adventure can also strip away the layers that disguise our essence—our authentic Self. The really challenging experiences that take you out of your comfort zone enrich your existence by revealing your true identity, not who you think you are, but who you *actually* are. These challenges open you up to endless possibilities by leaving you with a greater sense of self-confidence for having conquered them.

In the aftermath of the excitement, your senses are sharpened—you see, hear, taste and smell things more clearly. Everything looks more vibrant. Essentially, you become more alive. You've stepped into the realm of the unknown and emerged a winner.

The unknown keeps us growing. It shows us where our fears and limits are. It entices us to step out of complacency. If you don't step across the threshold of what you already know into the world of challenges, you never truly measure yourself. When you're in a challenging or dangerous situation and the wrong move can be a serious mistake (for us this is true when we're climbing), you automatically become totally present. The chatter and the noise of the rat race of your daily life stops and you move into a state of expanded awareness, open to the mystery of possibility.

"The most beautiful experience we can have is the mysterious.
It is the fundamental emotion that stands at the cradle of true art
and true science. Whoever does not know it and can no longer wonder,
no longer marvel, is as good as dead, and his eyes are dimmed."

—ALBERT EINSTEIN

We're not saying that the only way to expand your state of awareness is by doing something so dangerous it could cause you bodily harm. Pursue adventure at your own level. The endeavor will help you get to know yourself and explore who you are and who you can become. Happiness comes along for the ride; depression cannot exist in the excitement and absorption of the moment.

Study after study has shown that exercise is a remarkable aid for depression, as well as for a host of other diseases, from fibromyalgia to heart disease. It also bolsters cognitive abilities and self-esteem. Neurologically, exercise encourages nerves to grow and branch out, to communicate with one another. Regular exercise is also powerful ammo in combating the effects of aging—it helps improve muscle tone, strength, coordination and balance, and it helps strengthen bones. Still need more motivation to move your body? Lower levels of exercise have been related to lower levels of testosterone (yes, women need it too) and that leads to a lower libido. Need we say more? Go out and get yourself some exercise and adventure!

Mariel: I suffered from depression for most of my life until quite recently, and my solace and relief always came from exercising out in the wild. My connection to Nature has always been a friend and confidant for me. I have used and continue to use movement as a way to feel myself. Along with finding a way of eating that is balanced and pure, I have been able to completely free myself from mood disorders by exercise, laughter and healthy eating. I believe there are other non-toxic modalities that also promote a balanced brain. The one that has been most effective for me is Brain State Optimization, a method of balancing the brain hemispheres through sound therapy (www.brainstatetechnology.com). But the foundation of Nature, healthy food, exercise and fun are reasons I have arrived at a state of complete well-being in my life. Personally, I believe that we treat far too many mental illnesses with drugs rather than with the natural resources available to us.

My grandfather, Ernest Hemingway, was an iconic adventurer. He'd go out into the wild to fish and hike and hunt big game. He loved the feeling of coming face to face with an elephant, to box, and run with the bulls. He loved the danger and unpredictability

*of Nature. It was a way to face death, which is like facing your-
self. It seems that men particularly want to do this. There is a
belief that you lose yourself and find yourself at the same time
when you're in extreme situations and all your senses become
heightened. I believe this is where my grandfather was at his best.*

Take It Outside

At this point, we don't need to tell you that moving our bodies and
being out in Nature are as much a part of our lives as breathing. We
also like subjecting ourselves to new and invigorating circumstances—
we both crave adventure. It makes sense then that we prefer our
adventures to be outdoors. Moving around, getting our muscles working and our heart rates up while surrounded by a beautiful landscape
or seascape, is our ideal scenario. That raw, real, physical experience
of being at one with a rock when we're climbing or of succumbing to
a wave as we tumble inside it cuts through any mental clutter and
brings us back to the immediacy of the moment, back to our authentic Self. In any endeavor, whether it's physical, spiritual or cerebral,
the edge is the gateway to a breakthrough.

You'll find that the joy of the adventure and the confidence it
imparts envelopes you and gives you new tools for dealing with day-
to-day life. Stuck in a traffic jam? So what. Waiter forgot your water
after three requests? Not a life-threatening condition. The calm that
follows the rush of adventure becomes a more integrated part of you,
a reference point that you can return to as you encounter the stresses
of a hectic world.

Find Your Edge . . . and Your Confidence

We understand that the word "adventure" means different things to
different people. Maybe adventure to you is a long walk through the
city or a park by yourself, observing people, nature and the actions
around you. Or it could be taking your family on a road trip to a
national park with an unscheduled stop for a dip in the river. Whether
it's jumping out of a plane, riding horses, rock climbing, playing a

sport or maybe salsa dancing . . . whatever it may be, the point is that you are connecting with yourself—propelling yourself out of your comfortable cocoon and into an unfamiliar place that requires you to use all your senses to persevere. You can't find that edge unless you challenge yourself to a stroll outside your comfort zone.

Mariel: Before I met Bobby, I was hesitant to challenge myself or stop on road trips to do something random and off schedule. I was programmed to stay within my plans. During my childhood, if I kept order and control over everything I did, then I felt safe. That pattern continued into adulthood. Bobby never had that pattern. He was all about spontaneity, curiosity and adventure . . . still is today. Ever since we met, Bobby has ignored my worries over changing plans and has stopped dozens of times when we're on the road to check out cliffs and trees, canyons or caves. Even if we said we would be home by 2 o'clock and we ended up arriving home by 7 o'clock, he defied my rules of time. At first I found it super difficult, but after several road trips, now I welcome his spontaneous curiosity. It has happily even sparked my own.

Now that I allow things to happen more organically, I do things that are more physically challenging, and that gives me confidence. When I feel confident physically, it carries over to other areas of my life. For example, when I'm on a difficult rock face and I'm not sure that I'll make it, but I make a move anyway and I succeed, the boost in confidence I get is mirrored in my life. I now have a feeling of inner ease, like "I'm just here. I'm good."

Bobby: Free soloing (where you climb without any ropes) is one place where I believe I tap into a form of simple consciousness. There are hidden meanings in our existence, and a door opens up to this place of calm when we go beyond our unconscious limitations. There becomes a knowing without knowing what's coming. Human beings want to feel alive! It is this aliveness that gives us a purpose. We want to feel deeply. When I engage in anything intense, I find this calm and it becomes a form of spirituality. Adventure pushes us outside what we think we're capable of, outside of who we believe we are, and we become infinitely more than that.

*Nature is a manifestation of the universe and we are inherently
nature. So step outside what you believe to be yourself, and become
infinitely more than that because you already are.*

The greatest benefit of this demanding kind of adventure is that it
awakens dormant capabilities; it isn't just a fleeting experience. The
expansion in awareness you undergo as you face your fears and succeed (or even as you face your fears and fail) stays with you as you
return to your everyday walking around life. You dared to face uncer-
tainty, a great unknown; whatever the outcome, there is a release.
You'll feel a greater confidence in everything you do.

This confidence will have a ripple effect throughout your life,
enabling you to grow exponentially. You will recognize and use more
of your potential, become more alive. You'll have more courage to
tackle the things that used to stop you. Any fears will be minimized.
You'll know in your heart that you are bigger than any problem in
your path and will be able to work through them with more grace.
It's a lot of fun when you see your own growth and transformation.
Life becomes an adventure.

Mind-Body-Spirit Connection

Respect your body. It's your home as long as you're here.

These days virtually everyone recognizes that there's a connection
between the body, the mind and the spirit and that for optimal health
to be achieved, all have to be in balance. Many medical centers and hos-
pitals are adding mind-body facilities to help with diagnosis and recov-
ery. There's a yoga studio on every corner. But *knowing* and *feeling* are
two different things. To fully understand the idea of the integration of
the physical and nonphysical, we have to experience it. Exercise and
adventure help us synchronize the trinity of mind, body and spirit. Like
other endeavors we've spoken about in this book, exercise and adventure are tools we can use to reveal and understand our authentic Self.
Being fully aware of the relationship between every aspect of the Self
allows us to become stronger and healthier with more overall confidence.

Mariel: I tend to be clumsy and needed to become more conscious of my feet. So I began doing a mindful practice we call "aware stepping." This essentially means being aware of where my body is at any given time—what my feet are doing at every moment, what's around me, what I'm stepping on, and basically trying not to trip or bump into things. When I go out each morning to walk, hike or run, I'm much more present now. I'm not looking for it to be over quickly like I used to. I am aware of my body mechanics and posture as I move. With this physical awareness, there is an increased consciousness, which in turn adds to my awareness. And with that awareness I am more at peace.

When you exercise, do it mindfully and with intention. Feel each movement and be fully in your body. Use your mind to direct and observe what you're doing. Pay attention to every aspect of doing what you're doing in that very moment. If you are in your body and nowhere else, you are totally without thought, just present. After the adventure or exercise, take a moment to be still and let the activity resonate on a nonphysical plane. Be thankful for it; absorb it into your spirit.

Awareness is the stepping-stone to wisdom, and wisdom is the ticket to enduring everything that comes your way. With wisdom, you're better able to enjoy the highs and ride through the low times without getting swept away by either tide.

Start Moving Now

Pain is weakness leaving your body.

It doesn't matter how old you are, anytime (by which we really mean NOW!) is a good time to start moving your behind! Results are guaranteed. As soon as you start moving, your body starts changing for the better. And with your newfound awareness, that movement in concert with intention means you will achieve definitive results. When you move with awareness, the body responds in kind. You want to see the results of your efforts in running, walking or sports, right? Then do it with full focus—the result is that you are thinner, stronger or more agile. Whatever your intent is, it will be manifested physically.

Exercise ignites your hormones and gets your lymph system moving and your heart pumping. Our metabolism seems to slow as we age, or does it? We believe that people's habits change with age, leading to a more sluggish metabolism. They drive everywhere, walk less, play less, move far less than they did when they were young and energetic. Many of the signs we attribute to aging are only the result of a person's lack of movement and poor nutrition. Two studies from the University of Colorado's Center for Physical Activity, Disease Prevention and Aging found that older men and women can keep their metabolism just as high as young people . . . if they stay active. Exercise revs our metabolism up again.

Young people are getting "old people" diseases as a result of obesity, bad nutrition and a stationary lifestyle. According to the journal *Pediatrics,* half of overweight teens and almost two-thirds of obese adolescents have one or more risk factors for heart disease, such as diabetes, high blood pressure or high levels of bad cholesterol. We aren't helping the situation when our schools cut phys-ed classes due to budget constraints. And with all the video games, television, DVDs and computer technology, our children are spending more and more time in front of an electronic box instead of moving their bodies. Bodies need motion to be healthy. Health is freedom, as anyone who has lost his or hers will tell you. It's your responsibility to preserve your health the best you can.

Stay away from saying *used to:* "I used to play ball . . . I used to run . . . I used to do yoga." The *used to* statement is a sad commentary on what you could still be enjoying every day. Become an *I can do it* person: "I can play ball . . . I can practice yoga . . . I can run . . . in fact, I can sprint!"

Bobby: So many people say to me, "You know, I'm older—my metabolism has changed." My response is: "No, you have changed. You no longer get outside, ride your bike to your friend's house, spend most of the day outside. You sit while driving a car. You sit at a desk at work, and you sit and watch TV. After sitting for only 20 minutes, your digestion shuts down 80 percent. Your metabolism didn't change; your activity level did."

Get honest with yourself and see where you can move rather than sit. Stand up when you can while using a computer. Watch far less television. Get out and bike instead of driving where you can. Make time to run, jump and break some physical boundaries. It will shift you back into being a kid again.

There is a childlike wonder and awe living in all of us.

Good Form

It's important to learn good form before starting a new exercise. You want to strengthen the areas that need strengthening and coordinate your movements in a properly functioning way. It's no fun to move around if you're in pain. You've probably seen people running down the road, their knees barely rising because their hip flexors are so locked that they propel themselves by moving from their calves. Do that long enough and it will lead to painful knee injuries and ankle, hip and lower back problems. There goes the running.

Maintaining good form requires body awareness and focus. If you're starting a new sport or exercise, get advice from a pro before going all out. If your body's not used to the physical stresses of the sport, it may try to cheat, taking an easier shortcut when it's tired or in pain. This can lead to stress and imbalances that will turn into future disabilities down the line. During a weight-lifting exercise, instead of doing a full repetition of a movement, you may find yourself doing a half or quarter. You might use your hands to help get yourself up a hill to take the weight off your legs. It's better to do less weight and shorter duration of the exercise or movement correctly than to carry on beyond your limit doing it incorrectly.

Acknowledge where you are and be respectful of your body.

Bobby: For every kind of sport, training or playing, I give it everything I have. I leave it all on the field, on the mat, in the water, on the track, on the bike, in the mountains, or on the wall. Mentally I'm drained; emotionally I'm done. But spiritually I'm awake, and physically I smile.

Mariel: William Broad's book The Science of Yoga *talks about both the benefits and the dangers of yoga and how some people are getting hurt doing it. Like any movement practice, yoga has prescribed alignment and proper form. There are many variations on that form just as there are hurtful ways to do those postures and ways that are in alignment with proper body structure. All of it varies from person to person. Anything can hurt you if you don't start at the beginning and do it properly. Many people make the mistake of going to yoga classes that are above their physical and mental acumen. You must have a skilled and qualified teacher. If you are thinking of starting a new routine, make sure you are going to the best instructor you can find at a level that suits you. It's insurance for your future understanding and success.*

Walking with Eyes Closed Exercise

"Our eyes are not responsible when our minds do the seeing."

—PUBLILIUS SYRUS

One practice we've experimented with quite a bit to develop greater body awareness is walking with our eyes closed. Sound hard? You'd be surprised. We do this often when hiking. We close our eyes and try to find our way. Try this at first in your own backyard or someplace familiar to you. Obviously, you won't want to do this exercise near traffic, open water or other potentially dangerous areas.

You can begin by looking in the direction you want to go. Take note of where things are—a tree, a rock, a dip and so on. Then close your eyes and start walking. See how many steps you can take without peeking. Feel where the sun is, which way the breeze is blowing against your skin. Hear the sounds around you, insects or a plane overhead. Be aware of what your feet are touching. Listen to your inner sense of direction. See with your mind. Then open your eyes. Where did you end up? Try this for a few steps then 10, 20, 50, 100 steps to see where you end up. Counting helps you remember where you are and where you have been. Objects, sounds, shadows and light become familiar to you. Increase the steps as you go. The amount of time you practice will change as well when you become familiar with your surroundings and you begin to move faster with less effort.

We do this exercise with bare feet on hiking trails and along the shore to really feel the connection with the earth and put ourselves back in our bodies. When our feet feel the earth beneath us, we are more grounded, more in touch with our physicality and less cluttered mentally.

> *Mariel: I'm in my body much, much more now. While I've always been athletic and felt pretty connected, I was quite unaware of what my limbs were doing, as though they were separate from me. With awareness exercises, especially walking with my eyes closed, I've been amazed to see how much more of a connection I've gained. At first it was scary, and I peeked all the time even though I told Bobby my eyes were closed. With practice, I started to get a strong sense of knowing where I was without looking. I now realize how reliant I was on my sense of sight, and by closing my eyes it has heightened my other senses, enhancing my ability to hear, smell and feel things more easily. I feel like I've built a foundation of calm through being more observant, more conscious of my environment, and most importantly more present.*

Your body is your physical vehicle for moving through the world. Yet so many people live detached from it, experiencing much of life only with the mind. Computers and smart phones and other handheld devices compound the problem. We've become "humans thinking" and "humans doing" but not so much "humans being." Walking with your eyes closed is a powerful exercise for putting you back in your body, giving you a much more immediate experience of life.

Mix It Up and Make It Fun

We like to mix up our exercise. We'll go for a hike or a bike ride through the mountains or go climbing, surfing, paddling or swimming. Then some days we'll go to the track to run and we'll time each other. We help each other stretch, sometimes falling into each other for laughs. We play catch, wiffle ball and throw a Frisbee. And, as we talked about in Chapter 8, we love to go to school playgrounds and parks and use the swing sets and other equipment. It all involves tons of movement, hand-eye coordination and athleticism, and it provides a great workout even though it just feels like we're having a good time.

If you're bored with going solo, try a team sport that adds a social element to exercise. If you have the opportunity to play golf or tennis with a friend, or join a baseball or basketball team, it's a great way to get motivated to move, not to mention it's fun.

Look to your childhood for exercise and movement ideas. It's likely that the activities you enjoyed as a child are activities you would still enjoy today. You'll have a natural ability for them if you excelled at them in the past. Start carefully and slowly. If you're running, don't do a ten-mile loop your first day out. Acclimate your body; strengthen it rather than burn it out. And be realistic in your expectations: if you're not 20 years old, don't exercise as if you are. If you build slowly and consistently, you will come back strong and healthy. This is about being full of energy, reviving your enthusiasm for life and adding some flexibility to your mind and body. It's not about trying out for the Olympics.

Mariel: For years I worked out hard—always. I would start out with a new activity for half an hour one day, then the next day I would go for an hour, then the next day for an hour and a half, and the next day two hours, then two and a half hours and on and on, until I burned myself out, got sick and had to start all over again. It was like punishment, certainly not fun. So the idea that exercise is fun now has been a huge awakening for me. Whether it is walking, yoga, sprinting at the track or even going

to the gym, it can all be a place where laughter and silliness take
over. Even alone on a treadmill, I find a reason to smile and make
it a game.

As kids, many of us enjoyed exercise because it was fun. As adults, we have a knack for taking the fun out of the equation and soldiering on. Play again! Not only will it reconnect you to joy, but it will also reconnect you to your body and a higher level of fitness. The results are a healthier, happier and younger you.

Mix It Up at the Gym

We never regret when we go to the gym.
We only regret it when we don't.

We go to the gym together several times a week because we created our own gym in our backyard. It is not your average gym. It is more like a playground. As you have probably come to expect, we don't do the typical gym workout either. Instead, we try to find things to do that are more like play than punishment but still engage the body in a full workout. We'll use kettlebells, jump ropes, a slackline, rubber bands, pull-up bars, rings, parallel bars, a trampoline, heavy balls, climbing ladders, ropes, old tires, a climbing wall and large exercise balls and make up different ways to train and have fun at the same time.

Instead of what one typically does with the big gyro balls, we toss them to one another, seeing if we can do it back and forth 100 times. If we do, then we aim for 200 times. It always includes a lot of laughter, which, as we mentioned earlier, boosts hormone production and metabolism.

When we do the slackline, we play on it for hours, pretending we're tightrope walkers, turning six steps into the achievement of a lifetime and bowing to the applauding roar of our make-believe audience. Whatever we choose to do as "exercise," we approach it as if we are nine years old and playing a game. Before you know it, an hour has passed and it only felt like 10 minutes. We really work ourselves, but because it's so enjoyable, we aren't even noticing. When going to the gym is fun, when you really love it, you stick with it—and you naturally get better results.

Whether you experience your adventure and exercise in a gym, in your backyard, in the ocean or in the mountains, the thrill and the results are yours for the reaping. All you have to do is set aside the time and initiate the activity. When you find your edge in movement and adventure, the exhilaration, confidence and inner peace follow. Enjoy it!

POINT-EARNING ACTIVITIES CHECKLIST

ADVENTURE

- Tomorrow, before work, go for a run, walk or bike ride.
  If you already do this regularly, take a new route.   **10 POINTS**

- Mix up your gym routine. (If you don't belong to a gym,
  create one in your home.) Try two new machines or
  pieces of equipment. Toss a big ball back and forth with
  a friend and set a goal for how many tosses and returns
  you want to reach.   **10 POINTS**

- If you've got a dog, turn your daily walk into a creative
  exercise—do sprints (assuming your dog can keep up),
  then slow down, then pick your pace up again. Walk or
  jog backward. Hop on alternate legs! Try a bear crawl;
  you'll look strange, but who cares. By the way, you don't
  need a dog to do this.   **10 POINTS**

- Take an exercise class that's new to you—hip-hop,
  kung fu, tai chi, ballet, kettlebells, Pilates, whatever
  strikes your interest.   **10 POINTS**

- Make plans to try an activity that stretches your limits
  (but that is within range of your capability): dancing,
  climbing, trekking, water skiing. If you're afraid of
  heights, what about hot-air ballooning?   **10 POINTS**

- At the end of your next exercise stint, sit down for
  a few moments, close your eyes and let the experience
  sink in. Register and appreciate the mind-body-spirit
  connection.   **10 POINTS**

- Try walking with your eyes closed. Be safe—do this
  somewhere that doesn't involve cars, cliffs or potholed
  terrain. Take your shoes off and see how many steps
  you can take.   **10 POINTS**

- Play tennis with a friend, find a pickup basketball game
  or join a local sports league.   **10 POINTS**

- Revisit a sport or exercise that you enjoyed as a child
  and let it reignite your enthusiasm.   **10 POINTS**

- The next time you do your workout, whether at the
  gym or elsewhere, consciously make it fun! Exercise
  isn't a chore; it's an opportunity teeming with rewards. **10 POINTS**

- Make a bucket list. Write down anything you have ever
  wanted to do, every dream that you've had, from racing
  cars to flying planes to climbing mountains. Whatever
  it is, put it on your list, and do one or two of your
  bucket list items every year!   **25 POINTS**
                                                  for living your dream

                                    TOTAL POINTS _____

CHAPTER 10

BE MINDFUL IN YOUR RELATIONSHIPS

Relationships. They make up everything we do and everything about who we are. Think about it. We have relationships with everything we come in contact with, from the air we breathe and the ground we walk on to the way we perceive everything in our lives—it's all relationship. Our relationships with ourselves and to one another are the most profound game changers in this lifetime. All our relationships begin within ourselves and ripple out from there—family, friends, pets, neighbors, teachers, classmates, coaches. From the actions we take to the perceptions of everything we interact with, relationships determine our very existence.

We even have relationships with the plants in our garden that we nurture and help grow. In return, they provide us with beauty and life force energy. When it comes down to it, we have a relationship with *everything* in our entire universe. This connection to everything in our environment is critical to our human connection and paramount to our connection with ourselves. When we know how connected we are to everything, we realize every choice and every outcome affects countless relationships. From thoughts to food to water to plants to breathing to exercise and playing, we are creating who we are and how we are in the world. We are the outcome of every choice we make.

That said, to ensure healthy relationships with others, you have to embrace the guidance in Chapters 1 through 9. By bringing your most aware authentic Self into the equation of partnerships and friendships, you set them off on the right foot. By being healthy and physically active and facing your fears, taking responsibility for everything in your life, you exercise the muscles of your individuality—your relationship with you. When that is established, you're less likely to lose your Self within the context of a relationship with someone else.

As the ancient Greek philosopher Socrates advised: "Know thyself." This is the beginning. And then you will know everything because you are connected to everything. We have to be honest about who we are and how we show up in the world. Becoming our authentic Selves means positive personal growth and change is taking place. A genuinely healthy relationship with YOU carries over into balanced relationships with others. If you cannot love yourself, you can never love anything or anyone else. It's that simple.

> *Bobby: I change—hopefully every day—in order to grow and expand. I strive to be a greater human with a greater spirit, to love more and live life fully! Making mistakes and growing from them along the way, that is all part of the journey.*

The two of us are in love, and that is a gift we share. But without personal awareness, our relationship could easily fall out of balance and into the realm of codependency. We work daily to become more self-aware and conscious of our actions and thoughts. Relationship—how we relate to and with others—is a huge guide in anyone's life and brings out the best and the worst in a person, especially when the bonds of love and commitment are profound.

As a couple, we avoid criticism of one another by keeping our self-judgment in check. Relationships are about being truthful about who you are on every level so that you can be YOU.

> *Mariel: Relationships and love are very personal. When Bobby and I talk about food, we talk about how everyone is an individual, how each person finds the way of eating that suits him or her subject to their heritage, their genetics, their environment and their lifestyle. That's a private relationship as well. It is the same*

with how Bobby and I relate to one another. If we are choosing to live our lives in balance with nature and all the things we know to be true about healthy living (and we are), then together we are harmonious. What we choose to do, think, feel and say is mirrored in the choices we make, and the choices we make are mirrored in how we interact with one another.

Bobby: Want great relationships? Here are some principles I've learned to put into practice in my relationship with myself, others and the world around me. First, trust yourself, then go from there. I say break all the rules! Give what you want to receive in return. Show kindness to everyone. Work your ass off. Stay positive. If you fall down the stairs, simply say, "Wow, I got down those stairs fast!" Then get up and keep moving forward with positive actions. Define yourself, not others. If you love someone, tell them. Do not ever be afraid of failure. Before you give up, try it again and again and again and you will succeed! Always use your smile to change the world, and never let the world change your smile. Your dreams are an expression of your soul—follow them and you will live your life, not someone else's. Remember that there is always something to be thankful for.

Coming Together

When we met on a hike in the Santa Monica Mountains, the instant we glanced at one another there was this feeling of *I know you on so many levels*—in one split second. While we were hiking, there was a connection like we both knew we were home. Crazy, silly, laughing, knowing and being ourselves—that's how we were around each other. We shared so many of the same ideas and thoughts. It's that feeling of knowing that there is someone who gets you, that scares the hell out of you and excites you, all at the same time. When this happens, you probably should follow it. We knew we were friends for life no matter what. We had no idea how important we would be to each other in the years to come. Follow your heart; the rest of it will all fall into place.

It wasn't a coincidence that we met outside. Nature has always been a primary teacher for both of us. When you connect with Nature, you connect with yourself. To be individuals on the same path toward self-actualization in the great outdoors puts you in the present. When you are present, you can be with someone completely. That's how it happened for us. And we wouldn't have it any other way. It's a journey—always changing, always expanding! It's been one of the greatest rides of our lives . . . to be continued.

> *Mariel: I spent 24 years in a marriage where I belittled myself because that is how I saw my mother behave with my father. Regardless of my desire to be strong, independent and self-confident, I allowed myself to be less than I was because I thought that was what a woman did as a wife. I was married very young, and being fully honest with myself was too difficult. I was unaware of my inability to clearly confront how I felt. I don't blame anyone for how I was in my marriage, but now my awareness and intention to be myself is what motivates my life.*
>
> *When I met Bobby I was ready for a different kind of relationship. My years of codependence, fear and low self-esteem were coming to an end. I was becoming myself for the first time. In fact, I was happy to be myself by myself. When I met Bobby, he could see me for who I actually am, and I could see him in return. Though our relationship has its "moments," we are respectful of the pure independent Self that the other person is, and we encourage one another every day to take care of ourselves. I see and accept Bobby as he is, and he sees and respects me in return. I feel free and happy because of that.*

Stay Open for Dialogue

When you're comfortable in yourself, the natural, good-natured teasing that takes place in a relationship is accepted for what it is—a little fun! It can be instructive, too. If your partner is teasing you about spending too much time on the computer or on the phone or on a pet project, it might be worth considering whether the observation is justified. Are you tying yourself up with these things obsessively, maybe to avoid a conversation or something else that's more worthwhile? Maybe not, but see if there's room for calibrating the time you spend doing default activities—the ones that you do at the expense of others. Objectively speaking, is your partner right? Are you hiding from life by staring into a backlit screen?

If your partner asks for help while you're involved in a project, take a minute to weigh his or her immediate needs against yours. Rather than instantly feeling resentful that demands are being made on your time, consider the idea that in a relationship, some of your time is shared, like a joint bank account. Helping your partner may in fact be helping your relationship, and that pays dividends to you. We believe a good rule of thumb for maintaining balance in relationships is to invest 75 percent of your time and energy in yourself and 25 percent in the people around you. Your time is energy. However, that changes as life changes. Some days you give 100 percent to others and some days you keep 100 percent of your time and energy for your own needs.

Learn to Listen

As a couple, we work on practicing the art of listening to one another. Of course we're human and, like everyone else, are often in the habit of doing too many things at one time. Don't think we don't fight. We do. But we recognize the irritation or anger in one another for what it is and realize that it usually has to do with our own fear or something we are reacting to rather than responding to. We both take a step back and ask, "What am I doing to cause this?" Or the deeper question, "Who am I being right now?" Sometimes the answer is so clear that you are being your mother or father or you're reliving unconscious childhood stories that are no longer your reality. You are not being you in this moment. In those times, we know we have to pull ourselves out of the rush of day-to-day life or simply out of our heads to get back in touch with the present and our need to establish time devoted just to the two of us.

It's easy to run through your own thoughts even when your partner is speaking. You might think you're listening as you finish up that text or put the dishes away, but when you ask a question that's met with a hurt glance because your partner explained the answer several sentences ago, you might have to rethink your listening skills. Maybe you can't do several things well at once. Maybe you can put your fork down for a bit between bites and take in what your friend, lover or child is saying.

> *Mariel: My ego has taken a huge beating since being with Bobby. Because my "mothering" skills were so honed, I thought I could really listen while doing something else. Although I am female and multitasking is my nature, in relationships, I've learned a huge lesson. Ladies, when it comes to your male partner, if you are anything like me, I am sorry to say your man is not feeling heard. I have argued until I was blue in the face that I can listen fully while doing something else, but the truth is, I am not fully present with him when I am cleaning the sink focused on my Bon Ami, and it is disrespectful. I didn't like admitting this because I thought I was losing precious time for sink cleaning or getting rid of junk mail from my inbox.*
>
> *Now I take time to stop whatever I am doing and listen to Bobby, and you can't imagine how much love, appreciation and silliness I get in return. He usually tickles me and sometimes pretends to be a ballet dancer with the Bolshoi, complete with a Russian accent. It's ridiculous when a man of 200 pounds with muscles ripped like a racehorse points his toes and pirouettes from the hallway into the living room! Our relationship is teaching me daily how to listen and focus, and I am more connected. I feel a sweet humility when I am with this person who sees me so clearly, plus he gets to be seen and heard in return.*

Communicate and Discover

Obviously one of the keys to a successful relationship is the ability to communicate. This means relying on the self-awareness you've been cultivating and being conscious of your behavior together. The two of us are dedicated to being our authentic Selves and coming together as a couple while remaining individuals with two distinct voices. It makes for an interesting dynamic. We both have strong personalities, so there is a tendency to be competitive, but eventually we laugh about any disagreements and they are gone.

Bobby: I was raised in a neighborhood and family that used sarcasm all the time. I was brought up to believe that constant teasing makes you stronger. If you dared to be different, you were made fun of. Mariel could not be more different. When we first got together, my teasing made her cry. I have come to understand that just a small amount of teasing goes a long way. I don't need to make fun of her to win.

I am a guy from New York where sarcasm and irony is a way of life. When you're with your buddies, you win and you're right, even when you're not. My guy friends totally get that because that's the way we are. Girls typically are not built that way. Let me tell you something fellas, "win or lose" just isn't that important to them. Now I create space for both of us to win, laugh and be ourselves together.

I think George Carlin summed it up best: "Guys are stupid and women are crazy and women are crazy because guys are stupid." I make time to be with guys and to be a total idiot from time to time. Mariel gets together with her girlfriends to be girls, to talk about everything over and over again and to have fun and understand one another. Then we come back together. The key here is that just because I love Mariel doesn't mean she has to meet every one of my needs. Mariel is not a guy—thank God. I appreciate her and love her for who she is!

We make sure that when we talk about anything that has the potential for conflict, we do it when we are calm and not speaking through a haze of anger. We have become hypervigilant about addressing our "issues" almost immediately so that we can move through them and go on. We have a pact with each other: "I love you enough to be here honestly and show you your truth by not allowing your negative habits to continue." So far we are growing by leaps and bounds, although it means eating some humble pie occasionally. The payoff is a bigger and better Us.

Relationships are about finding our Selves as we discover another person. Through their eyes we might better see our own weaknesses, the limiting beliefs, the wounds and past traumas that are still affecting us today. Ideally, relationships allow us to confront our issues with support from our partner.

If a behavior or attitude or belief system isn't working anymore, if it's creating too much upset, anger or chaos in your life, a loving partner may help you pinpoint the problem. You can decide to change that behavior. Once you get that little bit of space between you and it, you can engage your self-awareness to say, "Okay, maybe I have a choice even though I didn't think I did." You can catch yourself just on the brink of the behavior and learn to pull yourself back.

Breathing is a first step to awareness here. When you feel anxiety or like you're ready to explode, take a deep breath in and exhale fully and ask your inner Self to guide you. Ask something like, "Help me to be present right now." Asking for presence after a deep breath pulls you into the moment, and you feel differently. If you are present, there really is no conflict; conflict arises in our attachment to either a story from the past or a desire for the future to look like something you are accustomed to. Ask to be okay with what is happening now and *know* that whatever you are feeling is fleeting. "This too shall pass" is a great phrase to remind yourself to stay here and not go forward or backward.

Mariel: There are times when I have to pull away from an old pattern. But now I have the awareness to see: "Oh, these are actually patterns, they're not the real me." I breathe and ask if what I am feeling is true in this moment. Trust me, sometimes I have to beg for guidance in difficult moments because the strength of my desire to be right or hold onto my old habits is strong. But when I take that space, I can pull away and get perspective. That is a huge growth in being present for me. I attribute my newfound self-awareness to the activities in this book. They have made a huge difference in my life and have given me the space I need to deal with my emotions more effectively when they show up.

Rocky Times Are Inevitable

Bobby: Guys need space. I am a guy who needs space, food, sleep, time to play and a chance to be physical every day. When I get these simple things, ask and I will do anything for you. Without them I can be difficult to be around. We all need different things in relationships. In general, men need to be heard and women need to be appreciated. But even this can vary from person to person. When we know one another's needs and can honor those, it helps prevent the conflict of relationships from taking over and diminishing the love that's there. Mariel and I choose to love, and the rest takes care of itself.

Sometimes when a partner voices his or her truth about something happening between you, it can sound like a criticism and can cause an unconscious reaction. If it comes from the right place, though— meaning if your partner is being genuine and delivering the truth from a place of love—see if you can take the information in as just that: information. On the other hand, if it becomes apparent that your partner is intentionally tearing you down and that the intention is coming from a place other than love, that is a valuable observation too. You may want to reassess the healthiness of your relationship.

Inevitably there will be rocky times in any partnership—romantic, platonic or familial. If you're frustrated or angry in one area of your life, it can seep into another area. It's okay to feel negative emotions, but be sure you know where they stem from so you can address them at the root rather than respond by lashing out at someone you love and who holds no responsibility for whatever's annoying you.

If you give your partner, friend or child the room to speak up for themselves in the moment, you avoid the buried bad feelings that can turn into long-lasting resentment. Listen. Challenge yourself to be quiet. Just listen and observe. Respond rather than react. *Response* has space around it and time to find presence. *Reaction* is explosive and emotional, not present. Listening gives you the ability to respond and accept.

Mariel: I allow Bobby to become softer and gentler. He comes from a background of teasing and fighting and being tough because that is how he survived. He lets that go with me because I am not a threat to him, so he is heard and seen as the gentle, kind and loving human being that he is. Just don't let his guy friends know. When I fully accept and hear him, I get the same in return. It's a good deal!

Bobby: Mariel used to be super emotional and reactive, and that came from years of feeling misunderstood and criticized. I see her. I don't judge her (unless I am judging myself), and when she feels seen, her emotional reaction time is cut in half. As men and women, we are always going to think and feel and process many things differently. That's what keeps the wonder, the journey and the mystery of the relationship continually expanding.

Keeping Your Self in the Relationship

Nobody can teach me who I am.

Relationships ask us to unveil ourselves to one another. In the process, we become freer as individuals, even as we're merging into a couple or a group of friends. Maintaining your individual sense of self while being involved with someone else is sometimes tricky. It's easy to slide into codependence—becoming obsessive about the needs of your partner at the expense of taking care of your own. Codependence doesn't serve anyone well. It's essential to learn to respect yourself and the other and to honor your independence and strength as well as theirs.

Take the time to connect with your authentic Self in all the ways we're advocating—through silence, meditation, food, ritual, movement, daily reflection and time alone. This will help you keep your identity within the context of your relationship. Both of us are extremely independent and very different, and yet we have a full understanding of each other. We know we're not the same and accept that that's okay. We love our differences. Although we love the same activities, we still love them as individuals. We tend toward different foods, we like different ways of moving into Nature, and we need alone time to be ourselves. Two whole people, both comfortable in their individuality, make a solid couple. The same is true for bonds with friends, family and colleagues.

This book is about how real and effective you can be, just by feeling your body, feeling your spirit and your connection. Can you accept that just being you is really enough? Can you find the courage to be you without an attachment to somebody else? Another person can validate your sense of Self without you having to give it away. Also, be sure that you look to validate yourself and that another's validation is simply gift, not something you need to define you.

The two of us don't *need* each other, but we do serve each other, and we bring each other up. A good relationship challenges you to be You first and to hold your own.

> *Mariel: I am emotional, and Bobby is practical and extremely masculine. It is the typical male-female dynamic—and one that I embrace. He is not me. I am not him. And I have no desire for him to change in any way. This is the first relationship where I am comfortable with the idea that as partners we are different. I love that he is such a man's man, that he has no ability to understand my sometimes crazy feminine emotions. He doesn't need to. Bobby and I have an underlying core belief system that orchestrates our paths together. Our unique differences make our union more special.*

Relationships offer us mirrors that reflect our qualities, showing us our strengths as well as where we are weak or scared, what our limitations are and where our belief systems may not work anymore. They can transform us. In films, as in life, the triumph of a character often comes through their relationship to someone else in the story who encourages them to persevere when they want to give up. By the end of the film, the character accomplishes something that otherwise would have eluded their grasp. The relationship was the fuel that led them to victory. Being connected to anyone on any level allows you to discover more about yourself.

Male/Female Energy

According to Hindu, American Indian and other philosophies, women represent the earth (Mother Earth) and men the sun. Certain traits align with the feminine energy and others with the masculine energy. The sun gives women energy to give birth, nurture and receive in the same way it gives the earth that energy to grow trees and plants that provide shade and food. Men are like fast-burning energy. Women are more tempered, slow and steady, and their energy is more long lasting.

Of course, these are generalizations and not meant to pigeonhole anyone into masculine and feminine stereotypes. What is undeniable, however, is the male/female energy, or dynamic, at work in the universe, and it is keenly visible in the context of relationships. A polarity takes place in the male/female relationship—this polarity is where the attraction to one another comes from. It's a dance between feminine and masculine energy. Rather than going into detail here about the differences between men and women, we simply want to affirm that where male/female differences exist, they can act as wonderful tools for growth in relationships when they are embraced and viewed as complementary.

Vive la Différence!

> *"Don't hate what you don't understand."*
>
> —JOHN LENNON

If the people you spent time with were just like you—thought like you, acted like you, experienced all of life from the same viewpoint as you—how boring would that be?! Thankfully, since no two people are exactly alike, we don't have to worry about that. What we must do, however, is learn to appreciate our differences rather than letting them become sticking points in our relationships.

One person in a relationship might be very routine-oriented and believe that life will fall apart without a schedule, while the other person may have a free-flowing, spontaneous spirit and feel suffocated when held to a tight schedule. This difference can either be a source of unending aggravation for them, or it can provide a great balance, eventually teaching one person how to be more flexible and the other how to add a bit of structure to their life. It's simply a question of how you both choose to deal with your differences—either with insistence that your way is the right way and the other must conform to it or with acceptance and open-mindedness.

Finding Space to Be Apart

Loving somebody doesn't mean you have to be with them 24 hours a day. Some people worry that if they spend time apart, they'll become disconnected. Granted, we don't recommend jetting off for a month at a time, but a day here or a weekend there can invigorate a relationship. Take some time to do something you love, maybe something that your partner doesn't enjoy so much. When you return, you bring back a sense of renewal and new stories from your trip and inject that freshness into your partnership.

Mariel: This has been an amazing learning curve for me, accepting that Bobby's not supposed to meet my every need. If he wants to go out and mountain-climb or surf, bike, run or swim with the guys, or be by himself, he goes. It took me a while, but now I like it when he's away; knowing he's fulfilled makes me feel good. I need my solo or girl time too, but for me to let go of him emotionally when he left was difficult at first. I had to trust that he wasn't going to leave me forever. That pattern was there because everyone in my childhood always left me. In my work on film sets, at the end of the shoot, everyone always left. Numerous suicides in my family reinforced the idea that people always leave. This relationship has helped me to deal with my abandonment issues, realizing they were not based in the truth of my life right now. Those patterns were holding me back and making me unhappy. Now I am thrilled to be alone and growing in my relationship with myself, plus I am super excited when we come back together again.

Bobby: Some people never settle down. We call them wild spirits.

Some might say I'm a wild spirit. Though I have had long-term relationships, I have never been married. I have my own take on relationships. In my view, two people don't have to be married to demonstrate amazing love for one another. For me love is patient and kind; it's willing to go through difficult times together and stick by the other person through all situations. Together we have the power to endure. Hope and faith, with moments of a perfect connection to one another, lifts our spirit. Love is all of these things; it's the energy of life itself!

Mariel and I spend a lot of time together. I sometimes say to her that I spend more time with her than I do with myself. At the same time, I can be alone with her because I can be myself with her. I still take time in Nature by myself, but I can also take that time with her and have space. We allow each other to simply be.

Be Realistic with Your Expectations

It's important not to put unrealistic expectations on your love relationship. No one person can provide you with everything you want or need. It takes a variety of relationships to meet all our needs. Friends, pets, children and mentors (academic, spiritual, running, gardening) are just a few of the relationships that can supply physical, emotional and spiritual needs not met by your significant other. Recognizing this is a big key to feeling happier and more satisfied in your primary relationship.

Relish your contrasts. Be excited by what you can learn from your partner's perspective. If your differences lead to a conflict, focus on response, not reaction. Reaction is guttural, instinctive and thoughtless. A response is mindful and considered and much more beneficial in communication.

Stay in the Present

"I am an old man," said Mark Twain, "and have known a great many troubles, but most of them never happened." So many things that we waste time worrying about never occur. We could put those moments to much better use by staying in the present and dealing with what's happening right now. There's no sense in wringing our hands over a future that we can't possibly know.

It's a helpful exercise to stay in the moment. Do what you're doing when you're doing it. Ease up on the multitasking. Don't call a friend while you fire up your computer and start surfing the Internet or while you're driving and having a back and forth with your GPS. If you're talking to a friend or spouse, to anyone, be there and nowhere else. If your child has popped into the kitchen while you're cooking, put the burner on low and sit down with him or her. See what's on his or her mind, what brought your child in to be near you. Make it your intent to really understand. Connection is the most important thing we have as humans, and the original instant message—face to face—is by far the most powerful.

It Starts With You

As we've been saying, relationships all begin with you. You set the tone, you set the parameters and you decide what is and isn't working. To do that effectively, you can use all the tools we've talked about in this book: connecting with Nature, finding and nourishing your physical body, eating and sleeping well and reconnecting with your center through meditation, writing, moving or silence. We think all these lessons are invaluable, but we also know that they need constant updating, like the software on a computer.

Sometimes the relationship you're in runs its course. If you're on a journey of self-discovery and your partner is not, maybe you've reached the end of the road together. That happens.

All of us are on our own journey through life. While many of our needs and circumstances are similar, they're wrapped in different guises and present themselves with varying intensity. Some of us have natural confidence but might have difficulty communicating. Others seem to be great at relationships, but a closer look will reveal that the bonds are forged at the expense of their own sense of self. All of us have to pay attention to our bodies, our minds and our spirits to be the best that we can be. When we are our best, we can bring that into our relationships and inspire others to be their best as well.

POINT-EARNING ACTIVITIES CHECKLIST

BE MINDFUL IN YOUR RELATIONSHIPS

- Check in with yourself when you get up. Remember that your relationship with your Self is the most important relationship of all.   **10 POINTS**

- The next time you're tempted to keep doing what you're doing when your partner starts speaking to you, stop and listen. Just listen.   **10 POINTS**

- The next time your partner does something that bothers you, step back and reconsider. Is it truly offensive or dangerous? If not, let it go.   **10 POINTS**

- If your partner, friend or any loved one seems upset about something you've done, take the time to understand their point of view.   **10 POINTS**

- Spend a full day not judging your partner. Accept him or her for who they are. Release the urge to "fix" them.   **10 POINTS**

- Be sure to express your love for your partner. Don't assume they know or feel it.   **10 POINTS**

- The next time tension arises in your relationship, address it quickly and from a place of calm.   **10 POINTS**

- When you're having a talk with your spouse or romantic partner, be present.   **10 POINTS**

- Make a list of five traits your soul mate has that balance some of your traits. Relish those differences. **10 POINTS**

- Make a list of five traits you have that are different from and help balance your soul mate.   **10 POINTS**

TOTAL POINTS _____

INDEX

ABOUT THE AUTHORS

Mariel Hemingway has written three best-selling books, *Finding My Balance, Mariel Hemingway's Healthy Living from the Inside Out* and *Mariel's Kitchen*. She is a passionate advocate for balanced living and mental health.

Mariel lives on Running with Nature Ranch in the Southern California mountains with her BFF (boyfriend forever) Bobby Williams, their two dogs Bindu and Tree, Mow the cat, nine beautiful hens, and a community of magical hummingbirds. She lives a life she loves in hopes of inspiring others to do the same.

Bobby Williams resides in the mountains of Southern California on Running with Nature Ranch that he created with girlfriend Mariel Hemingway. The stuntman/actor, adventurer, writer, health and wellness expert steps outside whenever he can. Bobby believes that by taking the seemingly impossible and making it possible, we tap into our unlimited human potential.

"There is always more sun in a day, and the best part of life is never knowing what happens next."

—BOBBY WILLIAMS

DISCARD